PRAISE FOR
MAKING FRIENDS WITH YOUR FERTILITY

'Friendly and practical, this book takes the reader on a journey from fertility basics and getting pregnant through to assisted conception, adoption and fostering. A must read both for single people and those in relationships, it looks at the difficulties that arise from secondary infertility and the fact that, sadly, treatment is not always successful. This book will be a robust, resilient friend for everyone considering their fertility, and an essential addition to any fertility professional's bookshelf.' **Susan Seenan, Chief Executive, Fertility Network UK**

'An important and illuminating book, not just for those struggling with fertility, but for anyone keen to better understand the emotional impact of having – or not having – children. **Making Friends with your Fertility** *is a book to read and absorb in stages and then return to. Grounded by tips and illustrations, it makes complex concepts really accessible. Simply brilliant.'* **Anya Sizer, Fertility Coach, Fertility Network UK**

'I will be sharing this book with my colleagues not only to share a brilliant and well-written piece of work, but also to share best practice for all healthcare professionals involved in fertility. Thank you Tracey and Sarah.' **Francesca Steyn, Head of Nursing, The Centre for Reproductive and Genetic Health**

'A very warm, informative and useful read for anyone exploring their fertility. Tracey and Sarah's book also provides an excellent resource for professionals who wish to gain more understanding of the emotional impact of trying to conceive.' **Freda Cuffe, Nurse Manager, The Lister Fertility Clinic**

PRAISE FOR *MAKING FRIENDS WITH ANXIETY*

'Simple, lucid advice on how to accept your anxiety.' **Matt Haig, Sunday Times bestselling author of *Reasons to Stay Alive***

'Sarah's advice is very sage. Deeply personal yet eminently practical, this accessible and engaging book should prove extremely helpful to anyone trying to cope with anxiety.' **Dr Ian Williams, GP and author**

'A self-help book packed with tips, exercises, and insights to ease worry and panic, this reads like chatting with an old friend; one with wit, wisdom and experience. Perfect for anyone suffering from this difficult disorder.' **The Book Doctor, Brighton and Hove Independent**

PRAISE FOR *SARAH RAYNER'S NOVELS*

'Brilliant... Warm and approachable.' **Essentials**

'Carefully crafted and empathetic.' **Sunday Times**

'A sympathetic insight into the causes and effects of mental ill-health as it affects ordinary people. Powerful.' **My Weekly**

'Explores an emotive subject with great sensitivity.' **Sunday Express**

'Delicious, big hearted, utterly addictive... irresistible.' **Marie Claire**

'A real page-turner... You'll want to inhale it in one breath.' **Easy Living**

'An irresistible novel about friendship, family and dealing with life's blows.'
Woman & Home

'Rayner's characters ring true, their concerns are realistic and their emotions guileless. Ripe for filming, this novel is both poignant and authentic.'
Kirkus Reviews

'Rayner's delicate, compassionate exploration of the struggles women face with fertility will resonate loud and clear with anyone struggling to have a family.'
Publishers Weekly

NON-FICTION BY SARAH RAYNER
Making Friends: A series of warm, supportive guides to help you on life's journey

Making Friends with Anxiety:
A warm, supportive little book to help ease worry and panic

More Making Friends with Anxiety:
A little book of creative activities to help reduce stress and worries

BY SARAH RAYNER AND DR PATRICK FITZGERALD

Making Friends with the Menopause:
A clear and comforting guide to support you as your body changes

Making Peace with End of Life:
A clear and comforting guide to help you live well to the last

BY SARAH RAYNER, KATE HARRISON AND DR PATRICK FITZGERALD

Making Peace with Depression:
A warm supportive little book to reduce distress and lift low mood

BY SARAH RAYNER AND PIA PASTERNACK

Making Peace with Divorce:
A warm, supportive guide to separating and starting anew

BY SARAH RAYNER AND JULES MILLER

Making Friends with Anxiety:
A Calming Colouring Book

NOVELS BY SARAH RAYNER

Another Night, Another Day
The Two Week Wait
One Moment, One Morning
Getting Even
The Other Half

TRACEY SAINSBURY
SARAH RAYNER

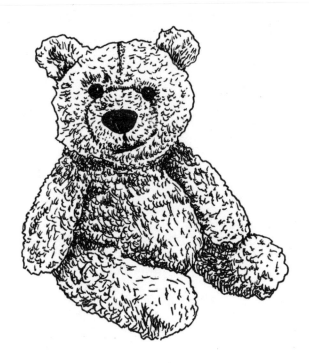

Making Friends
with your Fertility

A clear and comforting guide to reproductive health,
supporting you through the highs and lows of getting pregnant,
IVF and assisted conception, adoption, fostering and living child-free

Featuring illustrations by Sarah Rayner

This edition first published in 2018 by Creative Pumpkin Publishing,
an imprint of The Creative Pumpkin Ltd.,
5 Howard Terrace, Brighton, East Sussex, BN1 3TR.
www.creativepumpkinpublishing.com

Creative Pumpkin
Publishing

First Edition October 2017
Second Edition April 2018
Third Edition June 2019

ISBN: 9780995794856

Cover design and illustrations: © Sarah Rayner
Printed and bound in Great Britain by Clays Ltd, Elcograf S.p.A.

Publisher's Note

Making Friends with your Fertility provides information on a wide range
of health and medical matters, but is not intended as a substitute for
professional diagnosis. Any person with a condition or symptoms
requiring medical attention should consult a fully qualified practitioner or
therapist. While the advice and information in the book are believed to be
accurate and true at the time of going to press, neither of the authors can
accept any legal responsibility or liability for any errors or omissions that
may have been made, nor for any inaccuracies nor for any loss, harm or
injury that comes from following instructions or advice in this book.

FOREWORD

You will probably have received *Making Friends with your Fertility* from the team at the London Women's Clinic because you are a patient at one of our clinics or have attended one of our events. Alternatively, you may be a professional working with us. However you came by it, we hope you will find this book useful in understanding fertility and some of the most common techniques to help achieve pregnancy. We also hope that it will provide support through the process – and beyond – if treatment does not work out. Tracey, the author of this book, is part of our family at the London Women's Clinic – she is Senior Fertility Counsellor for the LWC Group – and we are proud to have her working with us.

At the London Women's Clinic we strive to provide affordable, accessible and effective fertility treatment across the UK, in a safe and supportive environment. You can read more about our clinics on pages 180-182. In addition, our free, frequent and popular seminars, open days and fertility fairs around the country allow people to make decisions about their treatment and their next steps on their journey with us. We understand that infertility can be hard, so we provide patient counselling at all our centres from Registered Fertility Counsellors, like Tracey, as well as monthly support groups and special events for single women seeking extra support through treatment.

I'd be delighted if you would share *Making Friends with your Fertility* with your friends, family and colleagues. At the LWC we are keen to provide essential advice to those with fertility issues and arm those who perhaps haven't yet thought through their own situations in depth yet – maybe because they're still relatively young, or not in a committed relationship. By producing bespoke copies of the book we hope that more people will benefit from Tracey and Sarah's advice and support: I hope you enjoy reading it.

Dr Kamal Ahuja
Scientific and Managing Director
The London Women's Clinic

Hello and Welcome

Maybe you're a woman reading this because you are trying to conceive or you're wondering if egg freezing can future-proof your fertility, or maybe you're a man who, alarmed by recent press reports[1] of falling global fertility rates is concerned about his sperm count. Or perhaps your partner is struggling to become pregnant and you want to understand more about her fertility, so you can say and do the right thing. No matter what your reasons for wanting to learn more, *Making Friends with your Fertility* is here to help.

One in six couples[2] can face difficulties conceiving, but this book is not just for those trying to have a baby. You could be the mum or dad of a daughter who has just started her periods – a parent keen to help separate fact from fiction. Or you could be the friend or relative of someone trying to conceive, keen to offer practical support. In short, **it's for everyone wanting to know more about fertility and conception, and the emotional impact of having – or not having – children.**

Making Friends with your Fertility is the guide I wish *I'd* had, a knowledgeable and compassionate 'friend' who is at your side (or, more literally, in your handbag or rucksack) to help you understand what's happening and support you. Unlike some friends, this

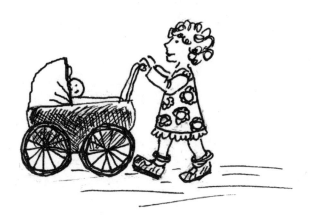

companion asks for nothing in return and can be picked up and put down at will. As you read there will be no awkward silences and, if you're considering conceiving, don't worry – there will not be so much as a hint that you 'just need to relax'. Because if I'd a penny for every time some well-meaning person said that to me over the years, my piggy bank would be full to bursting, and I appreciate how galling it can be!

About me, Tracey Sainsbury

For many women, conscious awareness of our own fertility often starts when we have our first period, but before that we often experience a less conscious maternal desire, and I was no exception. From as far back as I can remember I yearned to become a mum; I'd bathe my dolls with tender loving care, dress them with painstaking attention to detail and push them around in prams only months after I'd learned to walk myself.

My desires took shape as I grew, and by the time I was 14 I had firm plans: I'd meet 'the one' and we'd have our family – three boys, if you please – each conceived during very romantic love-making, of course.

The best laid plans don't always go to order, however. My periods started *way* before I was ready to have them, just before my ninth birthday – a hideous experience as no one quite believed they were here to stay, including me. I was taken to the doctor who said that as I had not shown other signs of early puberty, it might just be a one off. But stay they did, regular as clockwork for the next twenty years, frustratingly *just* until I started trying to conceive. Oh, the irony! Having spent years trying to prevent a pregnancy, my attempts to get pregnant continually failed. The more I tried and failed, the more determined I grew; I became a woman on a mission to have children, and left no avenue unexplored in a bid to do so. If my hormones were tested once they were tested twenty times, if a specialist suggested supplements then I'd digest them by the bucketful, and over the course of the next few years I must have peed on every brand of ovulation predictor known to womankind. As for sex – who needed to make love? – making *babies* was the order of the day. It left me feeling bored, barren and emotionally battered, but eventually, thanks to adoption and fostering, I *did* become a mother and, finally, the dream was real.

I'm at the other end of the maternal journey now; benefitting from my co-author Sarah Rayner's *Making Friends with the Menopause* book, and working full-time as a Senior Fertility Counsellor at the London Women's Clinic Group.

I have amassed around 20 years' experience working and volunteering with fertility-related charities and clinics including Fertility Network UK and the Lister Fertility Clinic. I was also on the Executive Committee of the British Infertility Counselling Association, a member of the committee for the National Infertility Awareness Campaign (now Fertility Fairness) and a member of the Human Fertilisation & Embryology Authority's National Donation Strategy Group.

Whilst the result of all this experience is that these days I'm something of an expert on fertility, the truth is that for most of us it remains something of a mystery – surprising given we quite literally wouldn't be here without it! It's hard to say where this gap in our knowledge stems from – perhaps we were taught badly in school, possibly it's the result of misrepresentation in the media. Certainly myths abound, so I was thrilled when Sarah asked me to co-write *Making Friends with your Fertility*. And talking of Sarah, this seems a good point to introduce her more fully.

About Sarah Rayner

Sarah Rayner is the author of five novels including the international bestseller, *One Moment, One Morning*. We met in 2011 when she contacted me about its follow-up, *The Two Week Wait*[3], which is about two women, each desperate to have a baby.

'I was in advertising back then, and it was writing copy for the London Women's Clinic that inspired me to write the novel,' Sarah explains. 'I read lots of case histories and found them incredibly moving, and thought my readers might find the same. In *The Two Week Wait* one woman donates her eggs to the other to subsidize her own treatment – and Tracey helped me get the emotional nuances right. I tend to get totally immersed in my characters, so whilst I've not had IVF or tried egg-sharing myself, fertility remains a subject I am extremely passionate about.'

More recently Sarah has published several self-help books, including *Making Friends with Anxiety* and *Making Friends with the Menopause*. 'The series aims to provide clear and comforting guidance on those mental and physical health issues many people find hard to talk about,' says Sarah. 'Fertility – and infertility – definitely fall into that category, and one day I had a brainwave: who better to ask to co-write a book on the subject I was so passionate about than Tracey? I emailed and within minutes she responded to say "Yes!"'

So that, in a nutshell, is who we are, and we've already touched on who you, dear reader, might be. Next, allow us to give more detail on *Making Friends with your Fertility*.

About this book
There are plenty of books out there on fertility, many of them good, so why read this one in particular?

1. It's short and it's simple
Unlike some weightier tomes, *Making Friends with your Fertility* isn't especially long or detailed. This is deliberate; we know how overwhelming the subjects of reproductive health and assisted fertility can seem. So instead this book aims to work as a practical 'primer', giving you an overview. We won't promise to answer every single question you might have on female or male fertility – there simply isn't room – and we'd invite you to explore any area of particular interest to you further. (The digital version contains links throughout, the paperback has footnotes, and both have a list of further reading at the end.) But by combining my knowledge with Sarah's writing skills, we hope to bust some of the misconceptions

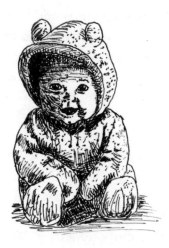

(if you'll forgive the pun) surrounding the subject of fertility, so you gain a better understanding of how it relates to your body both now and in the future.

2. Understanding fertility can help you, your family, and friends – a lot
We've already mentioned that one in six couples may have trouble conceiving, but this figure only relates to the number of heterosexual couples who experience infertility as conception has not occurred naturally. Fertility can be a source of interest or a cause for concern for *any* woman or man. Assisted conception and egg freezing are available for single women and women in lesbian relationships, and surrogacy is an option for gay men, too.

Whatever your particular circumstance, we believe ignorance is *not* bliss: knowledge can be empowering. We're also aware that sometimes a picture can speak a thousand words, so the text is offset by Sarah's illustrations and, where relevant, diagrams. We hope this combination makes for clearer communication and a more enjoyable read.

3. This book is written with honesty
That said, we haven't sugar-coated the facts: not everyone reading this book who *wants* to conceive, *will* do. Thus as we review the different methods of assisted conception, we will also be exploring the implications of our fertility choices, acknowledging the arguments and conflicts that take place consciously – and unconsciously.

4. Infertility can be isolating

We hope that understanding more will help you to feel less isolated and the tips shared will form the beginnings of a tool box of strategies to dip into, to help you to manage difficult times. We will also be signposting further resources so you can widen your support network and feel less alone.

5. This book isn't one of those 'be positive' books

Negativity is OK - in fact, it's appropriate. Neither Sarah nor I believe that humans have magic powers. We can't end a pregnancy simply by wishing it away, nor can we get pregnant as a result of positive thinking at the time of ovulation. We'd even go so far as to say that to encourage you to have extremely positive thoughts if you're trying to conceive can be just as angst-creating. Our hope is that once you understand more, you'll see you're not alone in finding fertility issues emotionally difficult to navigate, and wherever you are in the journey, there is nothing 'wrong' with feeling up or down, or both. By the end of this book we hope you'll be able to be kinder to yourself – however you are feeling.

6. Infertility doesn't just affect one person

Women trying to conceive are often in many relationships; sometimes with a partner, though not always, but also with parents, other family members, friends and colleagues. And if you're using assisted conception, you'll have relationships with professionals too. Our hope is that this book will help you to understand how you change within those relationships, how others can better understand you too.

7. We'll touch upon all the options, because there's more than IVF

Some people want to try to conceive at home, others in clinics with less or more intervention. So together we will explore the treatment options available, and how you can help yourself become fit for fertility.

We will also look at donor conception and donating eggs, sperm, or embryos, and briefly look at the UK regulatory framework and

NICE Fertility Guidelines. The frustrations often encountered when hoping for assisted conception funded by the NHS will be something we'll talk about too.

8. IVF isn't always successful
Contrary to media suggestion that IVF always delivers twins, the current UK national success rate for IVF is around 26%. We will explore alternate nurturing options, including self-nurture, and share more understanding of the healing process consciously and unconsciously as we embrace a different life than was planned.

9. Some people want more than one child, or two or even three... and sometimes more!
Secondary infertility can, for some people, have more of an impact than primary. If an oft-imagined fantasy included having three boys (that was my perfect family) and a son is born to the parent(s) in question, friends and relations can all too easily suggest that particular mother 'should be grateful' for the family she has, especially if she went through fertility treatment to conceive in the first place. But – oh dear – there's nothing like a bit of collective judgement to create a sense of guilt and shame, is there? Never mind that she'd like another, not just for herself but as a sibling for her firstborn.

We hope we will help any mum or dad experiencing secondary infertility to have a little more self-compassion as we gain more understanding about thoughts and feelings. We will also share insights so that anyone who knows someone experiencing secondary infertility can be proactively supportive.

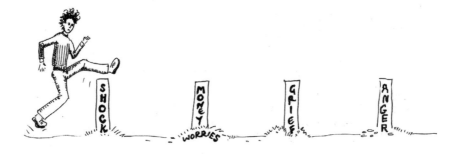

10. Peer support doesn't end when you finish this book

Sarah and the authors of the other books in the *Making Friends* series recognize that whilst books are fabulous tools for self-help, *people* bring the content to life. Each and every one of you reading this will have your own personal experience. No one person will have exactly the same physical or emotional response to the issues surrounding fertility, and we all have different questions and needs for support. For that reason, we have set up a group on Facebook, also called *Making Friends with your Fertility*. It's for anyone thinking about their fertility and exploring fertility issues or trying to conceive. The group is 'closed' to keep discussion private, so posts are only visible to other members, but you can ask to join at **facebook.com/groups/makingfriendswithyourfertility**. Please note that it is moderated by Admins in their spare time – not a doctor or fertility specialist (or me, or Sarah, though we will pop in regularly) so talking, even in this group, should not replace a clinical consultation.

Like a good friend, neither Sarah nor I have all the answers. A tip that might work a treat for one person might not work so well for another, but please trust that we will be with you in spirit as you read whatever you decide to do – or not do. Whatever the outcome is, we both wish you all the best on your fertility journey.

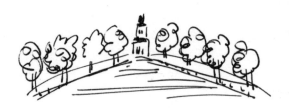

CONTENTS

1. **'F' is for Facts about Human Fertility**
   To start our journey we'll explore the fertility basics, looking at where it all begins with our hormones, eggs and sperm:
   - An overview of the main fertility-related hormones
     - Gonadotropins – in women
     - Gonadotropins – in men
     - Sex hormones
     - Other fertility hormones
   - Menstruation or periods
     - Problems with the menstrual cycle
     - Sanitary protection
   - Ovaries and eggs
     - Inside the ovary
     - More about eggs
   - Testicles and Sperm
     - Testes
     - Testicles
     - Sperm

2. **'E' is for Egg Meets Sperm – making babies**
   This chapter focuses on the stuff people do initially, i.e. without the need for intervention/assisted conception and thus includes:
   - Sexual Intercourse
   - Orgasm
   - Home insemination
   - An overview of pregnancy and its stages
   - Birth and the first few weeks
   - Men and non-birthing mums
   - Now you are three

3. 'R' is for Readying Yourself – self-care and lifestyle

Again, a general chapter for everyone trying to conceive: the dos, don'ts and don't do too much, for:
- Diet and nutrition
  - Here's the philosophy
  - What about special fertility diets?
- Exercise
  - Yoga and Pilates
  - Swimming
  - Walking
- Alternative therapies
  - Working with your body
  - More time
  - Finding a reputable practitioner
  - Acupuncture
  - Chinese herbal medicine
  - Mindfulness
  - Reflexology
  - Hypnotherapy

4. 'T' is for Time to Get Help – when making a baby is not so straightforward

Let's examine problems with fertility/those seeking assistance with conception in more detail:
- Reasons for seeking assistance with conception
  - Pregnancy loss
  - Being single and keen to have a baby
  - Being gay and keen to have a baby
  - Infertility as a medical condition
- Where to get help and what to expect
  - Making friends with your GP
  - Testing your fertility hormones
  - Additional fertility tests – for women
  - Additional fertility tests – for men
  - Support with tests
  - NHS or private?
- Fertility clinics
  - Choosing a clinic - regulations, rules, and ratings

5. **'I' is for IVF and Other Forms of Assisted Conception**
   A basic guide to the different ways that fertility specialists can help us to achieve a pregnancy:
   - Fertility Treatment
     - Timed sexual intercourse
     - IUI
     - IVF
     - Egg and embryo freezing
     - ICSI
     - IMSI
     - Donor conception as a recipient, a donor, or both
     - Surrogacy
   - Trying again
     - After unsuccessful treatment
     - Trying again after pregnancy loss
     - Secondary infertility
     - Trying again with donor conception

6. **'L' is for Loss – the emotional impact of fertility treatment**
   Here we take a look at understanding ourselves when we're trying to conceive:
   - Nurturing Capacity – Understanding Emptiness
   - Fantasy Loss Ownership - going with the FLO
   - Understanding the lows: Trauma and Loss
   - Understanding the highs: Hope and Excitement
   - Forget CBT, let's talk DBT

7. **'I' is for Involving Others – your relationships with other people**
   This chapter looks at why when we're 'just' trying to have a baby, no one else appears to understand:
   - Fantasy Loss Ownership – FLO in relationships
   - Hedgehogs: becoming prickle aware
   - Coping with other people's pregnancies
   - Sharing information… or not

8. **'T' is for Throwing in the Towel – time to stop trying to conceive**
   If we reach a point where we're ready to stop, what does it feel like, what choices do we have? Here we'll dip a toe in and see what it's like:
   - Calling it a day with assisted conception
   - Coming to terms with not having your own child and looking at other options
   - Adoption
   - Fostering
   - Being child free vs child less

9. **'Y' is for You – finding your own way through**
   - Your stories
   - Making friends with 'your' fertility
   - Beyond fertility
   - And so, the end is here

Join the conversation
An explanation of acronyms associated with fertility
Endnotes
Useful websites
Recommended reading – books and articles
About the authors
The London Women's Clinic
Books by Sarah Rayner

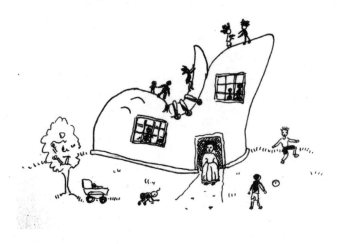

1. 'F' IS FOR FACTS ABOUT HUMAN FERTILITY

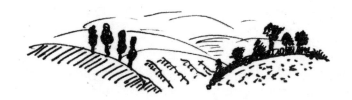

In the introduction I said that one of the aims of this book is to myth-bust some commonly held beliefs around fertility and trying to conceive, so we're going to start our journey together by looking at some facts about male and female fertility. This chapter won't get too technical, and is intended to 'set the scene' for the rest of the book.

So what exactly do we mean by 'Fertility'? As a broad definition, **fertility is the natural capability to produce offspring**, in the context of us as humans, anyway. It has other meanings – we also talk about 'soil fertility' and having a 'fertile imagination', for instance – but it's human reproductive fertility that we're focusing on here.

As you read on you may well come across aspects of the subject that you already know about, and others where your knowledge might be hazier. And because so many physical aspects of fertility are hidden out of sight and many people find it hard to talk about sex and intercourse, chances are you could learn much that's new.

It's a long time since either Sarah or I were at school, and whilst we're guessing you may well be younger than either of us and thus more familiar with sex education given you're reading this book, we don't want to assume you're an expert in human biology. Let's begin with a 'science bit' and look at what happens to us physically during our fertile years.

1.1 An overview of the main fertility-related hormones

Humans don't become fertile until they hit puberty, and women are no longer able to conceive naturally once they hit the menopause. These physical changes wouldn't happen without hormones. **Hormones are your body's chemical messengers which travel in your bloodstream to tissues or organs**. They're essential for everyday life – for digestion and growth, for mood control, and, in this case, for reproduction.

It's usually because of hormonal changes that we first become aware of our own fertility. Physical changes in our bodies can be seen as we sexually mature; girls begin to menstruate and develop breasts, boys have growth in their penis and testicles along with changes to their voice, which becomes deeper. Women can also develop fertility awareness if our hormones are playing up for one reason or another, and we encounter some sort of problem[4] such as irregular cycles, though for men there are often no visible symptoms.

'When I came off the pill to try to conceive, I noticed straight away how I changed during my monthly cycle. I found myself feeling sexy around ovulation, initiating sex, which I'd never done on the pill, and far less interested in making love towards the end, much to Drew's disappointment!' **Gita**

1.1i GONADOTROPINS – Hormones that stimulate the gonads in women

Sarah, like many people, thought 'gonads' a term for testicles, but actually, 'gonads' refers to both ovaries and testes, i.e. organs in the body that produce gametes, that's eggs and sperm to me and you!

- **Follicle Stimulating Hormone (FSH) is released by the pituitary gland**
  - It causes an egg to mature inside a follicle on an ovary
  - It stimulates the ovaries to release the hormone oestrogen

- **The pituitary gland also releases Luteinizing Hormone (LH)**
  - In the first part of a monthly cycle LH matures the eggs growing within the follicles. A surge in LH also causes ovulation to occur
  - In the second half of a monthly cycle, LH promotes the production of progesterone which is essential to support a pregnancy

TIP: The surge in Luteinizing Hormone is what is picked up by home ovulation kits. A test can notify you around 24-36 hours before ovulation so if you're trying to get pregnant it is the ideal time to – as Frank Sinatra would say – 'Make Whoopee'!

1.1ii GONADOTROPINS – hormones that stimulate the gonads in men

In women, hormone levels fluctuate during the monthly cycle – and we often know this to be true as they are marked by mood changes (though for me to call them 'mood changes' is something of an understatement – at times I felt almost like a different person). In men the rate of production remains the same (although I know many men – my husband included – who like to attribute their mood changes to hormones too).

- **Follicle Stimulating Hormone is released by the pituitary gland**
  - FSH causes sperm to be produced in the testicles, the two glands inside the scrotum that together are known as 'testicles' or, more informally, as 'balls'

- **The pituitary gland also releases Luteinizing Hormone**
  - This supports sperm development into mature sperm
  - It also stimulates the production of the male sex hormone testosterone

1.1iii SEX HORMONES - hormones that affect sexual functioning and desire

Both men and women produce the same sex hormones, in differing amounts. It's these hormones that give us our boy and girl traits. You may well have heard of oestrogen (sometimes referred to as 'estrogen'), progesterone and testosterone, but I am including dehydroisoandrosterone (even though it's quite a mouthful) here too. Specialists sometimes refer to it as 'the mother of all hormones' because it's essential for making our sex hormones. Some experts at the Centre for Reproduction in New York believe it can do even more and reduce – or even reverse – fertility ageing.[5]

> *'Mood changes – argh! I feel like Jekyll and Hyde, and yet we're trying to make a baby. My poor husband. Occasionally I wonder why we're still together – or rather why he puts up with me, as on some days **I've** had enough of me!'* **Jemima**

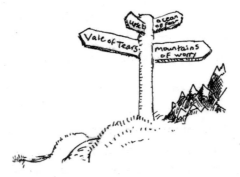

Sex Hormones in women
- **Oestrogen (E2) is produced by the ovaries**
  - It stops FSH being produced so that only one egg matures in each cycle

- It encourages the thickening the endometrium, the lining of the uterus in readiness to support a pregnancy
- It stimulates the pituitary gland to release the LH

- **The ovaries and adrenal gland produce testosterone (T)**
  - It helps in the production of oestrogen
  - It peaks just at the time of ovulation, increasing sex drive, then reduces dramatically after ovulation

FACT: Oestrogen and testosterone peak in the middle of a woman's menstrual cycle, which brings three changes; an increase in sexual desire, it becomes easier to reach orgasm and orgasms become more intense.

TIP: You might like to research when your own desire is at its peak. Much fun to be had, methinks!

- **Progesterone (P4) is released by the ovary, adrenal gland and the follicle itself**
  - The ovaries and adrenal gland produce most of the progesterone in women, but once the egg has been released the remaining collapsed follicle also produces progesterone
  - It maintains the lining of the uterus, called the endometrium during the middle part of the cycle and if pregnancy occurs promotes foetal development

- **Dehydroisoandrosterone (DHEA) - 'the mother of all hormones'**
  - The adrenal gland produces dehydroisoandrosterone which is essential to produce oestrogen and testosterone in both males and females
  - It might[6] help to improve egg quality in more mature women (over 35)
  - It might[7] improve sex drive in women

Sex Hormones in men

The production of sex hormones remains constant for men, so sex drive often remains constant too; this is one of the things we talk about a lot within fertility counselling, as the stress around not getting pregnant can result in a loss of sexual desire for both parties. This said, having your hormone levels checked by your GP can be a good first stop if you're not feeling in the mood at a time when there is pressure to perform.

> **FACT: You probably know that a low testosterone level suggests a low sperm count, but what you may not be aware of is that taking too *much* testosterone can also cause a low sperm count. This is why you should always speak to your GP or urologist[8] before taking hormones for fertility, and should only take those prescribed for you.**

- **Oestrogen (E2) is made from testosterone in men, a special enzyme helps some testosterone to change to become oestrogen**
  - It helps to regulate sperm development
  - It is important for sex drive and erectile function[9]

- **The testes and adrenal glands produce progesterone (P4)**
  - It helps sperm to function correctly
  - It helps sperm to fertilize an egg

1.1iv Other Fertility Hormones

There are a couple of other hormones that are important when it comes to your fertility; the first because it's the one test that is routinely requested ahead of a fertility clinic consultation and the second because (although most clinics often don't mention it, let alone test for it) the solution doesn't need a prescription and is free of charge.

- **Anti-Mullerian Hormone (AMH) is only produced in women**
  - It is secreted by the immature follicles inside each ovary
  - It thus gives an idea of the 'ovarian reserve' or 'egg reserve'; the higher the number, the higher the number of immature follicles
  - Is important because the amount of AMH indicates to a fertility specialist how we might respond to medication to stimulate our ovaries

- **Melatonin has an impact on both male and female fertility**
  - The pineal gland produces melatonin deep inside our brain
  - It regulates our body clock and too much or too little can affect our sex drive
  - It promotes healthy eggs in women and healthy sperm in men

TIP: Sleeping in a darkened room with no light and spending time outside during the day in natural light optimises melatonin production.

'Our sex life is always better on holiday. I assumed it was just being away until Freda mentioned reading about melatonin; we draw the curtains on holiday, but at home our bedroom is in the loft so we always look at the stars. I can really see the benefits of a better night's sleep, in addition to more frequent sex.' **Phil**

1.2 Menstruation or periods

When it comes to fertility, for many women menstruation is a double-edged sword. On one hand, the arrival of a period illustrates the completion of the menstrual cycle and the beginning of a new cycle of pregnancy potential. On the other hand, for me it was a crushing visible sign that – yet again – I *wasn't* pregnant. Little surprise, therefore, that if we're keen to start a family, our emotional response to having a period can be very mixed.

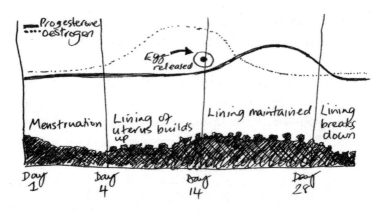

Hormone levels during the menstrual cycle

In medical terms, 'menstruation' is the shedding of the lining of the uterus, which, as I mentioned, is called the 'endometrium'. The cycle from one period starting to the next usually takes around 28 days. However, cycle length can range from 25-34 days and still be classed as regular. Mid-cycle the endometrium reaches the perfect depth to welcome an embryo. If pregnancy does not occur, then the endometrium begins to break down until hormonal changes trigger the start of a period.

Serotonin, a neurotransmitter, is a chemical produced in our brain which has many functions. Its effect on mood is well known, but what you may not appreciate is that the amounts women produce depends on the production of our other hormones, and these change throughout the menstrual cycle.

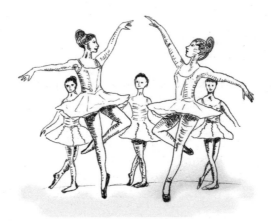

'What does that mean for me?' you might ask. Well, a doctor once told me that female hormones were like a ballet, with the dancers flowing in beautiful time. And for some women this is true; their hormones ebb and flow in perfect harmony, so mid-cycle, just when it's most useful, higher levels of oestrogen and testosterone, together with serotonin, promote a feel-good factor and increased sex drive. There are physical changes too; breasts often swell and cervical mucus takes on an egg-white consistency which is more sperm friendly. But if *my* hormones were a dance, they certainly weren't members of the Bolshoi – they were more like a troupe of toddlers, where everyone was out of sync and treading on each other's toes!

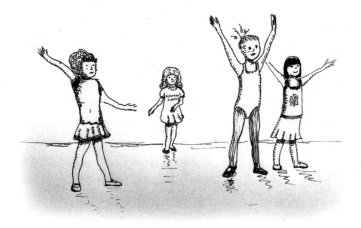

1.2i Problems with the menstrual cycle

Periods can be regular as clockwork, frustratingly irregular, heavy and clotty or light and clot free.

'I don't know where I am one month to the next.' **Janet**

'Bleeding problems are rarely mentioned. My periods are awful and my social life is suffering because of it.' **Theresa**

If you are concerned about your periods, please do speak to your GP. Sometimes their reassurance can be incredibly helpful.

- **Pre-Menstrual Tension or Premenstrual Syndrome (PMT or PMS)**
  There isn't a definitive known cause for PMT or PMS, but doctors think that there can be an increased sensitivity to the changes in the hormonal dance, with sufferers being more responsive to progesterone. Often symptoms include anxiety and sometimes depression too. If you're experiencing high levels of either, I strongly recommend reading Sarah's other books in the Making Friends series: *Making Friends with Anxiety* and/or *Making Friends with Depression* to gain insight and be introduced to a range of coping strategies.

- **Endometriosis – growth of the endometrium outside of the uterus**
  Endometriosis is a menstrual disorder which occurs when the cells that develop in the endometrium grow outside of the uterus. As well as impacting fertility by blocking or distorting the fallopian tubes and so preventing egg and sperm getting together, endometriosis can be extremely painful. Endometriosis UK[10] is an excellent resource for anyone who has, or who suspects they have, endometriosis.

- **Amenorrhoea – not having periods**
  If your periods haven't started by the age of 16, or you haven't had a period for a couple of months (and are not in the run up the menopause), the NHS advises that you see your GP. There can be many reasons why periods cease – including a change of diet and stress.

'My periods stopped for three months after our dog died. We don't have children and for me her death was heartbreaking.' **Sally**

Not having periods will impact on fertility if you are trying to conceive with your own eggs.

- **Dysmenorrhoea – painful periods**

  Dysmenorrhoea can be crippling, sometimes for an hour or two, sometimes much longer. I have counselled many women who have thought painful periods are normal and who have suffered for years, but often they have a treatable cause, so if you have very painful periods, please ask your GP to refer you for tests. One common cause of painful periods is fibroids. These are benign growths in the uterus that vary in size and, depending where they are positioned, may or may not impact on fertility.

- **Menorrhagia – heavy periods**

  Fibroids can also cause heavy menstrual bleeding, but sometimes periods can be heavy and there isn't a specific cause. Because fibroids can impact your fertility, if you are trying to conceive, it's well worth checking out the possibility with your GP.

> **FACT:** Not having regular periods does not always mean that you cannot achieve a pregnancy with your own eggs as medication can sometimes help. On the flip side, having regular periods does not always mean that you can achieve a pregnancy with your own eggs, as we don't always produce healthy eggs.

We will look more at reasons for not getting pregnant and the options available in Chapters 4 and 5.

1.2ii Sanitary protection

If you're considering fertility treatment, **you might be surprised to learn that women are often advised not to use tampons during treatment or afterwards if the treatment is not successful.** This is because the cotton in tampons causes a slight increase in the risk of infection.

If your heart sinks at the prospect of switching from tampons, I understand. Having started my periods at such a young age, my mum didn't feel it was right for me to use them. She was concerned that I might find them alarming, and believed they were 'new-fangled' anyway, so she stuck to what she knew – a very basic pad with loops that attached to a belt. The result is that I didn't use my first tampon until I was 17 years old, and I can still remember how wonderful it was to be freed from sanitary towels. So when I was trying to conceive, I too balked at the idea of going back to pads.

You might ask: 'If I can't use tampons, can I use a menstrual cup?[11]' and the answer is yes, you can. Joyce Harper, Head of Reproduction at University College London, assured me that medically there is no reason why not, although it is always important to be as hygienic as possible when using one.[12] Whilst I'm familiar with cups, I've not tried them myself as they've become popular since I stopped having periods. So I put a shout out on Twitter to find out what women thought about them.

'I couldn't use tampons due to repeated infections from changes in the PH of my body caused by using tampons. The Moon Cup is brilliant - I'll never go back to pads.' **Ellie**

'If you follow the (very comprehensive) instructions included in the packaging of the Diva Cup, then you shouldn't experience any discomfort, or worse, leaks. A heads up though is that you have to insert it horizontally, as opposed to vertically like a tampon. Another point to note, whilst it says the cup can be left inserted for up to 12 hours, I would advise that you empty it every 4-6 hours initially so you can understand your flow better and avoid the cup potentially overflowing.' **Jen**

Ellie and Jen were not alone: the response was wholly positive. There are many different makes and colours of menstrual cup, and all the brands come in different sizes for women who have previously given birth vaginally and those who haven't. Several women said they used a pad in addition if flow was heavy, just to be extra safe, but I always used to supplement a tampon with a pad on heavy days anyway, so don't see this as a negative.

TIP: Menstruation can be a timely reminder to engage in a bit of self-care, especially if we are trying to conceive. Try to make some space for *you*, and be more aware of your emotions.

And if you're not sure *where* you are at emotionally, don't worry – we'll be coming back to the subject in Chapter 4.

1.3 Ovaries and Eggs

Ovaries are the female reproductive organ that produces eggs.

FACT: An egg is the largest single cell in the human body. Each one is about as big as a grain of sand and is just visible to the naked eye.

Doctors often talk about 'oocytes' (pronounced 'oo-cytes' or 'O-O-cytes') or 'ovum' or 'ova'. All of these refer to the egg itself.

Egg development during the menstual cycle

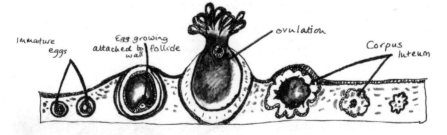

FACT: Although we are born with 1-2 million eggs, a process called Ovarian Follicle Atresia has been reabsorbing eggs since our mothers were around 20 weeks' pregnant. Talk about poor design – we have the most eggs we will ever have before we are born!

1.3i Inside the ovary

On Day One of the menstrual cycle, hormone changes cause a number of follicles to begin to grow. These fluid-filled follicles, known as Antral Follicles, can be seen on a pelvic ultrasound scan from around Day Three of our cycle. Usually, the increasing progesterone levels stop all but one of the follicles from developing further. Typically, a single follicle goes on to become mature, but non-identical twins or triplets are when more than one follicle develops or when a follicle has more than one egg inside.

As the follicle develops, the egg inside begins to mature too. It starts off attached to the wall of the follicle, then as it matures the luteinizing hormone causes it to release from the wall and bob about inside the follicular fluid. When the pressure inside the follicle reaches an optimum point, the follicle tears, expelling the fluid and the egg contained within. This is known as 'ovulation'.

Some women can *feel* when they ovulate. I only became aware of the sensation when we began tracking ovulation. As I came to be more tuned into my body, I noticed a mild, 'stitch-like' pain.

After ovulation, the egg heads off on an epic adventure: it is sucked in to the fallopian tubes and progresses towards the uterus, hoping to encounter a healthy sperm along the way.

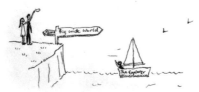

1.3ii More about eggs

In every human cell there is a pair of chromosomes. The female egg contains one half of each pair – the X chromosome.

> **FACT: The sex of a baby is determined by the status of the sperm. An X sperm will give a female child (XX) and a Y chromosome will result in a male (XY).**

The egg is surrounded by a cloud of small cells called, appropriately, a 'cumulus'. This acts like a system of locks and keys around the egg, allowing easy access for one sperm if the egg is healthy and stopping sperm wasting their time if it knows already that it doesn't have the potential to create a viable embryo. Each egg has the potential to be fertilized for around 24 hours following ovulation.

If the fallopian tube has been damaged in some way, perhaps as a result of disease within the tube itself, or due to a previous ectopic pregnancy or medical condition such as endometriosis, then the egg and sperm may not be able to meet in the tube and fertilization cannot occur.

You are probably well aware that egg quality and quantity decline with age. Neither will you be surprised to learn that this correlates with a higher chance of miscarriage or failure to conceive. Knowing something to be more likely doesn't prevent it being very upsetting if it happens to us, however, and we'll return to this subject in Chapter 6.

'I had four cycles of IVF, produced lots of eggs and embryos but I never got pregnant. We did genetic tests in our next cycle, none of the embryos we created were healthy; my doctor said at the time better not to conceive than to miscarry or have to make decisions about whether to carry on with an unhealthy pregnancy. At the time, I thought that was harsh, but thinking back she was probably trying to be helpful and probably right too.' **Claire**

Whilst the average age of menopause in the UK is 51, this is *only* an average, so it's hard to say that there is a 'normal' age for menopause. Most doctors consider menopause to be early if a woman's periods stop before she is 45, and this affects about 1 in 20 women[13]. For the ovaries to stop working altogether before the age of 40 is rare; this is known as Primary Premature Ovarian Failure (POF) and affects about 1 in 100 women. Secondary POF can occur as a result of medical treatment such as chemotherapy or an infection. If you're going through a premature menopause, you might find Sarah's book, *Making Friends with the Menopause*, useful. The Daisy

Network[14] is also an excellent resource – it's a large support group for women who've experienced a premature menopause.

If the egg reserve is depleted or there is a higher number of eggs but the quality is poor, that doesn't mean you can't carry a child however. Pregnancy is still a possibility with egg donation and we will look at this in more detail in Chapter 5.

1.4 Testicles and Sperm

1.4i Testes

The testes are the male reproductive organs that are contained in a sac hanging outside of the body behind the penis. The sac and testes are known together as 'testicles', and it's common for the two testicles to be slightly different in size. The testes begin to become active during puberty. When I was at school, the boys stood in line for a 'cough and drop check' with the school nurse, who would discreetly feel for a testis in each sac. My son didn't have a similar check however, as it is no longer considered appropriate. In my view this is a shame – it helped young men by giving them early reassurance all was normal, and made them more testicle-aware.

You might wonder why in all of evolution nature has designed a body part with such obviously enormous reproductive importance to hang off the body in such a vulnerable way. It's to do with temperature: should sperm get too hot, they lose potential for fertilising an egg.[15] To ensure excellent sperm production, the testes can respond to temperature. They shrink or retract when it's cold, and expand when it's warm.

However, there's a bigger factor in sperm production than heat – hormones. And so this chapter comes full circle, as we're back with luteinizing hormone triggering the testes to produce testosterone. And it's testosterone, together with follicle stimulating hormone, that activates sperm production.

1.4ii Testicles

In a recent article, Professor Allan Pacey of the University of Sheffield states[16] that, in simple terms, the bigger the testicles the better, because 'the bigger the factory, the bigger the quantity of sperm produced'. He says scientists also recommend that men ejaculate every two or three days to keep the reservoir of sperm in optimal condition.

Some men find it difficult to ejaculate inside a woman's vagina, but unfortunately this is not often talked about. If you have any concerns about ejaculation please don't suffer in silence – sometimes the testicles can contain blockages or enlarged veins which can affect the production or transport of the sperm so it's worth asking your GP if they can refer you to a urologist. Because they specialise in the urinary tract and male reproductive organs, he or she will hopefully be able to ascertain what is causing the problem.

The pressure to perform if you and your partner are pro-actively trying to conceive can also impact penile function.

TIP: Whilst ejaculation is essential if you are trying to conceive at home, it's worth pointing out that intercourse isn't.

When we explore conception in Chapter 2, we will look at suggestions for trying at home where intercourse is difficult.

If you've had a vasectomy in a previous relationship, then want to try for a family with a new partner, it's sometimes possible to have the procedure reversed.

'I tried to have my vasectomy reversed. Unfortunately it wasn't successful, but I am pleased we tried, or I would always be wondering what if...?' **James**

Alternatively, sperm can be surgically removed.

TIP: There are no guarantees that a reversal will work, but if you've had a vasectomy, it's worth asking your GP to refer you to a urologist to explore the best option for you.

1.4iii Sperm

It takes around 74 days for each new sperm to be created and every ejaculation typically contains millions of sperm. As the sperm are ejaculated, they mix with a fluid known as 'semen'. In any sperm sample, most of the substance will be semen.[17]

FACT: A sperm is the smallest cell in the body. It takes around 175,000 sperm to weigh the same as an egg!

So now we know how the right combination of hormones are to enable us to produce eggs and sperm, next we have to make sure we get them in the right place at the right time. It's this we'll look at next.

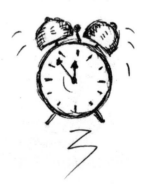

2. 'E' IS FOR EGG-MEETS-SPERM
MAKING BABIES

As we've just been exploring the basics of human fertility, it makes sense to continue our journey by looking at getting pregnant, and the physiology of making babies. In this chapter we'll run through a typical pregnancy; one that occurs when you do it the 'fun' way, i.e. without the intervention of other people (such as donors) or fertility treatment. Should you end up on the road of assisted conception and successfully conceive, the three stages of your pregnancy will be the same, so we do recommend you read this chapter whatever your baby-making circumstances.

Sexual intercourse within heterosexual relationships is one of the topics you may remember from school. Sarah recalls watching her father blush when she told him they were to discuss it in class, and I vividly recollect the letter home to prepare my parents, with my dad shaking his head and asking, 'Why do you need to know?' Doubtless similar reactions still prevail, although these days, schools often have a lesson for parents and guardians to help them answer their children's questions without such embarrassment.

There is often an assumption we all – women especially – understand pregnancy. What we didn't learn at school or from the adults who cared for us, we're supposed to have gleaned since from the internet, TV and magazines, with friends filling in any gaps in our knowledge. Yet my experience at Fertility Network revealed otherwise, where I provided regional and online support, advice and information. I've read hundreds of leaflets and articles, and found that much of what is written is hard to fathom. Even when it's explained verbally, information often seems shared too quickly or comes across as needlessly complex, or both, so I hope you find it helpful to go back here to the basics on getting pregnant.

We will look at:

- Intercourse and home insemination
- An overview of pregnancy from conception to birth
- Men and pregnancy

2.1 Sexual intercourse

The Oxford English Dictionary[18] defines sexual intercourse as 'sexual contact between individuals involving penetration, especially the insertion of the man's erect penis into the woman's vagina, typically culminating in orgasm and the ejaculation of semen.' Yet to me the very word 'intercourse' always sounds so prescriptive; it hardly conjures up beautiful love making with a soul mate, with the best orgasm ever, does it? As Sarah says, 'It's such a cold, dry word, it makes me go "ouch" to say it.'

We may cringe at the word and find it awkward to talk about, yet humans have been making babies through having intercourse since, well, humans came into being. It's been written about for hundreds of years – the Kama Sutra (including chapter 2, the infamous one about sexual harmony) was written over 2000 years ago, for instance. Yet even though many of us find some sexual positions more arousing than others, it has yet to be proved that any one position is more likely to promote pregnancy than another. So no matter if you choose to swing from the chandeliers or have sex missionary style, it won't make an iota of difference. Though the amount you do it can; **intercourse every 2-3 days is deemed to give the best chance of success.**[20]

The truth is that for most couples, the road to getting pregnant is sometimes fun, sometimes a chore, and very, very occasionally the earth might move for one (or, better still, both) of you. If a pregnancy is planned but you've not been trying for long, then it stands to reason that sex might well be enjoyable and regular, but if you've been trying for a long while, it can cause anxieties for both men and women.

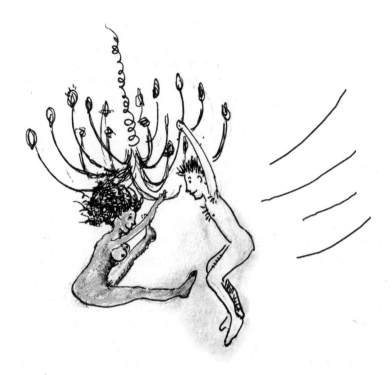

TIP: Don't forget to spend time focusing on intimacy. Yes, ejaculation is important, but so is mutual pleasure.

Remembering that you're in this together as a loving partnership can alleviate some of the stress, too.

2.1i Orgasm

There's conflicting research about the impact of female orgasm on conception. There's certainly no proof that orgasm *reduces* the chance of pregnancy, and one study suggests that being more sexually satisfied increases the frequency of intercourse and so increases the chance of the sperm and egg getting together.[21] So whilst there's not enough evidence to suggest having an orgasm is actively helpful, I wouldn't wish to discourage any woman from trying to climax if and when she can!

Having the penis ejaculate inside the vagina can sound simple, but for lots of reasons some couples find it difficult, if not impossible. Vaginismus[22] is **the term used to describe involuntary tightening of muscles around the vagina whenever penetration is attempted, and is** one medical condition which can impact greatly on a woman's ability to tolerate intercourse, for instance. Penile and ejaculation problems[23] such as erectile dysfunction can also prevent intercourse happening at the right time for fertilisation to occur.

2.1ii Home insemination

Home insemination isn't restricted to lesbian couples and single women, who may consider home insemination as a quick fix to get sperm from a known donor in to the right place at the right time; home insemination can be a great idea as a first step to assist conception if there's a problem with intercourse.

If you definitely don't want to be pregnant the rule is simple, always use contraception.

TIP: If you do want to get pregnant, there are a variety of home insemination devices available, of which the best known is *Stork*,[24] **which can help to have sperm in the right place at the right time. Whilst they won't increase the chance of a routine pregnancy, these can be very helpful when problems with intercourse occur.**

These home insemination devices may also help with common fertility difficulties including a low sperm count, sperm motility issues and unexplained infertility – subjects we'll return to in Chapter 4.

However you get it there, if a healthy sperm meets a healthy egg in the fallopian tube at the right time, fertilisation should occur. If it doesn't, please don't blame yourself – or your partner. As I've said before, we aren't powerful enough to prevent fertilisation occurring with our thoughts or feelings, so it's *not your fault.* Keep at it. And if fertilisation does occur, it's the start of a whole new adventure.

2.2 An overview of pregnancy – conception to birth

TIP: An NHS Bounty Pregnancy Information Pack is available to all pregnant women in the UK.[25] **It's full of practical advice and explains pregnancy in detail, week by week, as well as giving lots of factual information about birth and family life.**

You'll normally get your pack at your midwife booking-in appointment, so don't forget to ask your healthcare professional for yours. It won't answer your questions right now, however, so let's take a closer look at the three stages of pregnancy here.

2.2i First Trimester – 0-12 weeks

I always found it odd that pregnancy dates are measured from Day 1 of your last menstrual cycle – i.e. the day you found out that you *weren't* pregnant from the previous cycle, but that is how it works.

A full-term pregnancy takes around 40 weeks: two weeks 'preparation' and 38 weeks baby growing. This two-week preparation time is when our hormones are causing an egg to mature, ovulation to occur and the egg to be released into the fallopian tube.

> **FACT: The egg travels to the fallopian tube with the strongest pull, usually the one closest to the ovary we've ovulated from, but if a tube is blocked the egg may travel round the body to the tube on the opposite side.**

Fertilisation occurs when one sperm enters the egg. At this point, chemical changes make sure no more sperm can fertilise the egg.

If we were to look more closely down the microscope, after 24 hours we'd see a circle with two dimples in the middle. These are the DNA of the egg and sperm,[26] very much ready to begin to grow together, and at this stage the embryo is known as a *Zygote*.

Fertilized Egg

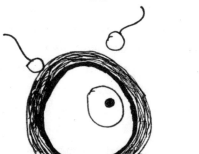

Zygote Embryo

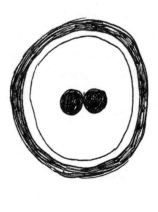

Week 3 sees the two dimples become two cells within the egg, then four, continually splitting to form more cells and expand in size; as the embryo reaches the uterus the cells will have evolved to become what I affectionately call 'the blobby bit' and 'the bobbly bit'. The more technical term for the blobby bit is *Inner Cell Mass* – it's this that will grow in to the baby. The bobbly bit is the *Trophoblast*, which will become the placenta, and together they form a *Blastocyst Embryo*.

Once inside the uterus, the egg shell becomes too small to hold the expanding embryo and it hatches out from the shell to implant in to the lining of the uterus, the endometrium.

Blastocyst Embryo

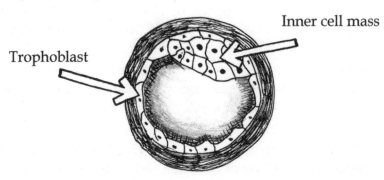

Inner cell mass

Trophoblast

When the embryo implants some women experience a discharge or blood spotting.[27] When I was trying to conceive I was told to look out for this and remember developing a bit of a discharge obsession. I later discovered that this behaviour is common in women who are trying to conceive and even has its own acronym 'FKC' which shouldn't be confused with KFC as it stands for *Frequent Knicker Checker*! Should you find yourself similarly fixated, rest assured you are not alone.

> *'I thought John hadn't noticed my increasingly frequent trips to the loo, but eventually he confronted me, concerned that I had a bladder infection. When I explained I was checking my knickers and I'd be happy to see blood if it was day 20-24 but gutted if it was later as it would most likely be my period, he totally got it.'* **Sal**

By Week 5 you will have noticed that your period hasn't arrived as expected, although cramping as your body adjusts can sometimes feel like the onset of period pains, which can be confusing. This early in a pregnancy, if you take a home pregnancy test or have a test with your GP, it can confirm a pregnancy, but the results aren't necessarily conclusive. If your test is negative but after a few days your period still doesn't arrive, do another test. If you're still worried, please speak to your GP. They can explore other reasons why your period might not have started.

> *'Every month I hoped we were pregnant, then came the cramps. I'd got so used to the pattern that when the cramps came again, I assumed it was my period, and I had even had a bit of spotting which I thought meant it was a bit earlier than usual. I simply assumed the stress of trying had sent my hormones haywire. My husband said "Trish, do a pregnancy test, just to check" as he thought I'd been a bit odd – and he was right. I was pregnant. He still teases me that I spent months obsessing yet he knew before I did!'* **Tricia**

Lots of exciting things happen between Weeks 4 and 8. For protection, the embryo grows within the amniotic sac surrounded by fluid. Here the essentials for life begin to take shape – the central nervous, breathing and digestive systems all develop, and a hollow conduit called the *neural tube* is formed which develops into the brain and spine.

If you have an internal scan at Week 6, you might see a heartbeat. At this point the growing baby appears a bit like a tadpole; the bump at the end is the head developing as the brain begins growing within, and arms and legs can just be made out as small buds. These grow fingers and toes which start off with webbing in-between.

By Week 9 your embryo is now a foetus, growing at 1mm per day. Your uterus will have doubled in size since implantation, to be about as big as a lemon. The changes within can promote physical changes in a 'mum-to-be' too. Tiredness is really common, as are sore breasts and an increased need to pee.

Having missed a couple of periods, it's time to make an appointment with your GP or local midwifery service, if you've not already done so, so that your antenatal care can begin.

'I thought I'd pop to the doctors to let my GP know I was pregnant and I'd be in and out in no time. I wasn't prepared for the number of questions; my health history and my partner's too, along with general questions about how I was feeling. I assumed this had become my booking-in appointment, but no, that was even more epic! That appointment took nearly two hours. Though I'm not complaining – I felt special and really cared for.' **Fiona**

By the end of the first trimester, the foetus is more human in appearance, though, at around 2.5 inches/6cm, still very small. All of the skeletal structure is present, but it's soft and pliable because at this stage it's made of cartilage, which hardens over time to form bones, some of which fuse together to become stronger.

Towards the end of the first trimester you'll have a 'dating scan'.[28] In addition to checking that everything is as it should be, this will provide confirmation of your due date and possibly a photo too.

'When we said that we didn't want to know if I was expecting a boy or a girl the sonographer looked surprised. She put a big sticker on my notes not to tell us, as apparently it was very obvious. She didn't say, "obviously that's a penis!" or "obviously there's no penis!" so thankfully we were none the wiser.' **Aretta**

FACT: It's important to note that not all pregnancies result in a positive outcome. Sadly, one in four pregnancies routinely ends in miscarriage.

We'll return to the subject of Pregnancy Loss in Chapter 4.

2.2ii Second Trimester – 13-27 weeks

The second trimester sees the foetus complete its development and begin to grow, putting on weight, getting stronger and more equipped to survive on the outside.

With your body adapting well to growing your baby, the symptoms of pregnancy can become more manageable. If you've experienced either feeling sick or vomiting then this often subsides and eventually stops.

'Actually, I don't think I did feel better, it's just that feeling permanently tired and needing a loo close by became normal. That said, as my bump became much more obvious I felt less self-conscious about needing to explain myself, and that was a relief.' **Chloe**

Your foetus will have been moving for some weeks, but as there's plenty of fluid and room to manoeuvre most women aren't normally aware of their baby changing position until midway through the second trimester. After this it's often much more noticeable, and sometimes you might feel their hiccups, too.

TIP: Antenatal classes[29] can help you meet other local parents-to-be and provide help and support. The National Childbirth Trust is the largest provider of antenatal care, but other local classes may be available too, so do ask your midwife what's available.

By the end of the second trimester, the foetus is over 30cm in length, a similar size to a large cauliflower, weighing around 1kg. The baby might spend most of its time tucked in the fetal position, but for me the most magical thing about this time is that relationships begin to form within your family, as the foetus starts to recognize your voice... and that of your partner.

When we adopted, I wanted to discover more about what children's experiences might be like before they are born, so I attended a *pre-birth attachment workshop*. The brain scans of each pregnant woman and their unborn babies were shown as their partners began to speak. To see the brains of the mums light up showing cognitive processing taking place and their babies' brains light in the same way was amazing, but once the babies got to 27 weeks old something even more incredible happened: there was a delay while the baby 'checked' with their mum, showing they were thinking *is this the right way to respond?* before mirroring. It was beautiful to see these early attachments, and for me only reinforced how important it is to feel emotionally well-supported during pregnancy. It's OK to be anxious or stressed at this time but experiments like these suggest that stressing about stress might well make a baby anxious too. On the other hand, if we're stressed and manage it well, we teach a growing baby that difficulties are manageable and provide reassurance before birth, helping them to develop resilience.[30]

TIP: The NHS, your Midwife or GP can provide or direct you to resources for emotional support during pregnancy.[31] You might like to note that if you are one of the many women who experience depression during pregnancy, the PANDAS foundation is an excellent source of support, along with Sarah's other book in the Making Friends[32] series: *Making Friends with Depression*.

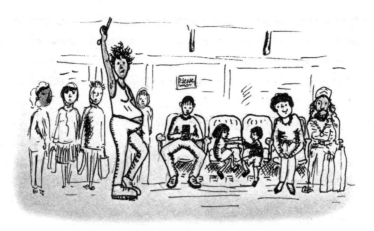

By the time you get to the end of your second trimester, the foetus is fully formed, so if you were to deliver prematurely, there's a good chance your baby would be able to survive, with medical support.

2.2iii Third Trimester – 28-40 weeks

The third trimester is often the one that feels the quickest. Given that delivery can routinely take place any time after week 37 that's not surprising – it's often several weeks shorter than the first two.
Your baby continues to grow in size. The senses develop – they hear more and feel more, and their eyes open. You'll be more aware of them physically, too.

'At the start of the third trimester I loved being pregnant and felt fabulous. Then the tiredness, similar to the first few weeks returned, along with fat, swollen ankles and horrendous heartburn. And in the last couple of weeks as my baby began to turn in readiness for his escape, I felt like a washing machine.' **Dyta**

TIP: Although you might have lots of things planned for your maternity leave, I always suggest holding off on making plans until you finish work, as you won't know how you're going to feel until you get there.

There are often more frequent antenatal appointments as delivery day approaches, some of which may not be planned. You want to be able to play it this time by ear.

2.3 Birth and the first few weeks

Attending antenatal appointments and a regular local antenatal class should give you the opportunity to learn about the different birthing options[33] available. You can consider if you would like a home or hospital delivery, and discover more about birthing centres, which are run by midwives. You can also think about if you'd like a water birth or natural delivery, and so on.

TIP: Making *a birth plan*[34] with your partner or birthing companion can be a great help, and should include everything about your ideal birth. But it should be etched in pencil, not set in stone. You'll want to be able to adapt it moment by moment, and don't feel bad if you end up not sticking to it. As long as you and your baby remain safe, wherever possible your wishes will be adhered to.

The birth itself and the early days of parenting are different for everyone, but here are some of the tips I've heard over the years that have proved particularly helpful:

- **If someone offers help, say yes**, even if it takes a while to think of what they can do.
- **If you can't think what someone can do, ask them to cook you a meal** that can be frozen and reheated by simply putting it in the microwave. You can never have too many ready-to-go-meals in the freezer, it's a fact!
- **A home baked cake is always welcome**, especially during a night feed.

- **Organise a short-term cleaner or ask for help with housework**. If someone can take a load of washing home and return it, ironed, it can be a godsend
- **If there's someone you trust with your baby, ask them to hold or watch the baby so you and your partner can _both_ have a day-time nap.**
- **If you have pets, planning ahead can be a really good idea.**[35] It may seem easier to have a dog out of the house, but pets need to get used to your new addition too.
- **Have two nappy change/outing bags, packed and ready to go.** Then if someone suggests an outing and if you're in the mood to say yes, you won't have to get things together and can simply head straight off.
- If you decide to express milk so that a partner, professional help or a good friend can help with feeds, **hire an NHS grade double-expressing milk pump**. I'd advise you to opt for the same model that you used in hospital, this will be much more effective than buying a home model off-the shelf, and could well end up cheaper too.[36]

So far in this chapter we've focused on what's going on for mum and her growing baby, but pregnancy is also a time for dads or non-birthing mums, so now let's take a closer look at some of the issues involved for them.

2.4 Men, non-birthing mums and pregnancy

When it comes to men about to become dads or women about to become mums with a pregnant partner, I often find myself frustrated because most of the guides, websites and apps seem to pigeonhole fathers or non-birthing mums dreadfully. Often, a second parent's role comes down to one thing: you are the main support for your now-pregnant partner. It's time to become more involved in cooking, cleaning, laundry and pampering – foot rubs, neck massages... you get the picture. And if I get irked, goodness knows how annoying it is to be a bloke or non-birthing mum reading this stuff!

Whilst I do know one man who was so delighted about the prospect of becoming a father that he virtually morphed into Mrs Mop overnight,[37] if you don't feel so mellow about it all, rest assured this is quite normal.

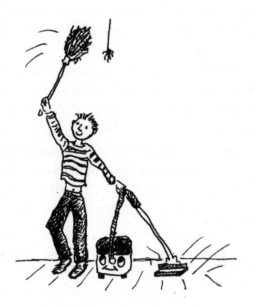

In my work with couples I've often found we end up talking with sadness at the loss of closeness in a relationship. Partners often mention they lack attention. As mum gazes downward at the bump, you might feel that eye contact with you is decreasing, and miffed if the bump receives an affectionate stroke which may have once been for you. A sense of guilt or shame or resentment is common; dads and non-birthing mums sometimes say they feel silly or stupid about this, especially if they were very keen to start a family too. But all these feelings are understandable; pregnancy means a huge change for both of you.

'Shirts, they were the thing that got me – Lucy had always taken pride in making sure I left in the morning looking well dressed. I cleaned our shoes, but she pressed my trousers and ironed my shirts – God I sound old! – but as the pregnancy progressed, it felt like she stopped caring about me. I wouldn't have minded, but I'm rubbish at ironing. When we finally had a row, which had been brewing for ages, Lucy suggested if I really wanted them doing I should take them to the dry cleaners. I know she had a point and ironing when she was heavily pregnant was a big ask so this all makes me sound like a prat, but it really got me down. I did try, but now we use an ironing service, and when Lucy is back at work we'll carry on using them. It's one less thing for us both to think about.' **Rob**

One of the biggest responses to pregnancy can be fear. This is an entirely appropriate reaction, especially to a first pregnancy. The cost of a baby in the first year alone is enough to make many younger people decide to delay parenthood to their thirties and beyond, and finance is not the only factor we can end up worrying about. What's going to happen if one of you is not working and progressing up the career ladder? Will the balance shift in your relationship as a result? Will you still manage to be a loving partner? And what about becoming a parent? Will you both be good enough? Sometimes the prospect of becoming a parent can promote reflection on our own experiences of being parented and bring up thoughts and feelings around the relationships we had and now have with our parents. Looked at like this, it's little surprise all these all worries can end up going round and round in our minds, making us very fearful indeed.

However you respond, please remember, **there is no right or wrong way to react.** Whilst talking about your feelings can help to keep both of you mentally well and happy, I appreciate it can be difficult, especially if you're not usually that open about your emotions.

TIP: Try not to beat yourself up. Honour and accept your responses, whatever they are, and talk them through as a couple if you can.

2.5 And now you are three

When your baby arrives, sometimes chatting becomes easier; there's a strong desire to discuss the new arrival and it can help to validate your relationship and make changes feel real. Becoming parents is a huge transition and taking time to get to know your baby together is important, so I'd advise you not to invite too many people round in the first few days and weeks you're at home. It can be unexpectedly exhausting, even if your baby sleeps well, and all too often both mum and dad can end up sleep deprived and irritable.

TIP: Making time for intimacy – not necessarily intercourse – is important throughout pregnancy.

Skin-on-skin contact helps you both to feel loved, cared for and supported; so hug lots and, even better, hug when you're naked! If you're tired and struggling to find time for intimacy, you might like to make showering together a regular part of your routine. We'll come back to the subject of intimacy in Chapter 7.

Having looked at making babies the fun way, just in case things aren't going to plan, let's have a look at additional steps you can take to optimise your fertility in our next chapter, 'Readying Yourself'.

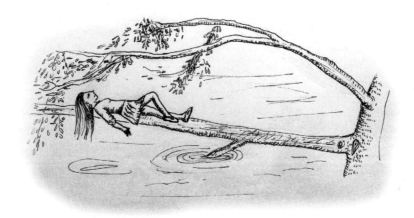

3. READYING YOURSELF
SELF-CARE AND LIFESTYLE

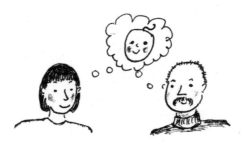

In Chapter 2 we looked at the basics of conception and pregnancy, a 'best case scenario' if you like, when fertilization occurs easily and naturally. But sometimes making a baby is not quite so straight forward. This was the case for me; in spite of diligently taking a pre-conception supplement[38] from the day we started trying, I didn't have any joy conceiving. After a few months I began to wonder if my husband and I were both in tip-top shape to make a baby. Was there anything more we could do to improve our chances of conceiving or to help us to cope better whilst we're trying? Here in this book, I thought it would be best to look into this before we explore medical intervention, but you may decide to investigate both together or go to your GP rather than exploring alternative therapies.

Whatever stage you're at on your journey, this chapter aims to give you some pointers. We'll look at what I wish I'd known – the dos, don'ts and don't-do-too-much-ofs in terms of:

- Diet and nutrition
- Exercise
- Alternative therapies

You can read it from start to finish now, or return to it later – it's totally up to you.

3.1 Diet and nutrition

At this point you could be forgiven for wincing, 'Ah-oh, here comes the hardcore diet plan.' Fear not. I think it would be unfair to suggest you follow a regime I couldn't undertake personally. So, I'm *not* going to insist that you stick to a rigid diet. I'm inclined to think a 'little bit of what you fancy' doesn't cause much harm, and Sarah has a similar philosophy – in truth both of us put this theory into practice perhaps rather too often! It's against this backdrop that we've written this section on fertility and nutrition.

3.1i Here's the philosophy

Making time to look after yourself isn't anything to feel *guilty* about. 'Keeping your body and mind healthy is not *that* different to making sure your car is serviced or your computer is backed-up,' says Sarah. 'I'd even go so far as to say that keeping yourself well is as much part of being a responsible, self-sufficient adult as other pursuits we often value more highly such as working hard or looking after others.' So how does this manifest itself in terms of what to eat?

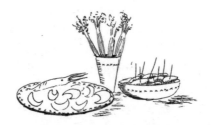

Do:
- **Minimise alcohol consumption.** The Chief Medical Officers for the UK suggest no alcohol at all when trying to get pregnant as it impacts on both male and female fertility. Alcohol can lower your body's ability to absorb calcium and can raise blood pressure too so if you drink, keep it to a glass a day.[39]

- **Cut back on caffeine.** Drink less coffee, tea and caffeinated soft drinks. (You should avoid <u>high-caffeine energy drinks</u> entirely.[40]) Caffeine causes your body to excrete calcium more quickly and speeds up your heart rate which increases blood pressure.
- **Reduce salt.** Like caffeine and alcohol, salty foods can cause you to lose calcium and speed bone loss, as well as intensifying hypertension. Processed and canned foods tend to be high in salt, so limit your intake. When you do eat these foods, look for low- or no-salt-added brands.
- **A good calcium intake** is important at all ages. You also need **a good supply of vitamin D** to help absorb calcium. You can get vitamin D from just a few minutes of sunlight and from fish, oysters, and packaged foods that have been fortified, such as cereal. A vitamin D supplement along with Folic Acid is suggested as being all you need to take in terms of supplements when trying to conceive.[41]

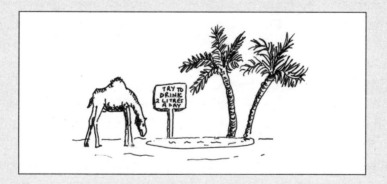

Don't
- **Succumb to diet/binge cycles** – this will cause great highs and lows in blood sugar and is likely to increase mood swings, irritability and anger.

- **Eat excessive sugar** as it limits your liver's ability to metabolize oestrogen and impairs the immune system[42] – avoiding processed foods is a good way to reduce your intake of sugar.
- **Eat excessive commercially-raised beef, pork and chicken** because these meats contain a high amount of saturated fats and decrease the body's ability to metabolize oestrogen.

3.1ii What about special fertility diets?

These days, social media seem awash with diets designed to help you conceive. Maybe it was ever thus; pineapples – that was the fad when I started trying to conceive many moons ago, before the days of Twitter. The main component in the stem is a substance called Bromelain, which it was said would boost the immune system and is a natural anti-inflammatory, thus would aid implantation. So I juiced dozens of pineapple stems – at least they were tasty – but still I didn't conceive. I'm sure that if juicing pineapple stems *did* increase the chance of a positive pregnancy test, all assisted conception units would insist on you eating or drinking pineapple…. They don't.

Since then it's emerged that there is no evidence to support Bromelain as a fertility drug,[43] and I'd advise that you avoid similar faddy diets. Instead, most nutritionists who specialise in fertility suggest taking a back-to-basics approach regarding pre-conception dietary planning. So, alongside the dos and don'ts above, **stick to whole foods, preferably organic, that are simply prepared**.

TIP: A colourful diet, rather than weighing and measuring or focusing on fat free, high protein or low carbohydrate is the best thing to aim for.

If we eat colourfully, every meal will include a higher number of fruits or vegetables than if we are eating mainly bland foods. Look at your plate – if a savoury meal is mainly beige, brown, white or cream, throw in some carrots or beetroot or sweetcorn.

In addition, **a healthy BMI[44] can promote fertility**. Being over or underweight can impact on the production of some of our hormones or how we respond to them, so working out what is a healthy BMI for your height and working towards that can be helpful.

TIP: Accessing support from people who are trying to lose or gain weight for the same reason as you might help you to reach your goal weight quicker. Some of the online weight-focused forums have a section for fertility, and some of the fertility forums include sections for weight issues.[45] And don't forget that our *Making Friends with your Fertility* Facebook group may also be a great source of support on all matters including weight loss or gain whilst trying to conceive.

> **FACT: All women trying to conceive are advised to take folic acid and vitamin D.[46]**

You can choose to take a pregnancy all-in-one supplement or pill if preferred, but there's no evidence they will be more beneficial than simple folic acid and vitamin D for promoting a healthy pregnancy or boosting fertility in general.

For men, some studies[47] have shown an improvement in sperm quality and/or quantity after taking an antioxidant supplement, but there's no validated study to support their use in women.

For women, especially mature women, one study suggests an increased chance of success with assisted conception if Dehydroisoandrosterone (DHEA, a naturally occurring hormone that decreases with age[48]) is taken, but this is not yet considered to be enough evidence for it to be used routinely when trying to boost fertility and DHEA supplements are not routinely available in the UK.

3.2 Exercise

If you're using exercise as a way to promote a healthy BMI then great, carry on – I don't want to be the one who stops you. However, when thinking about fertility, you might think *all* exercise is great, and thus I'm going to tell anyone who isn't exercising regularly to get in training for a marathon, now. In fact, a Norwegian study[49] found that hard workouts where you train to the point of exhaustion can impact your menstrual cycle, which in turn will impact fertility. If you're not having regular periods, you're not in with a regular chance of conceiving, end of. So **don't continue with anything that seems to be interfering with your menstrual cycle.**

If you're having or planning assisted conception treatment, speak to your doctor, as some high impact exercises may present a risk of twisting in ovaries that are being or have been stimulated.

These two caveats aside, thinking holistically (i.e. in terms of you as a whole person), some exercise is often really helpful. If you've been

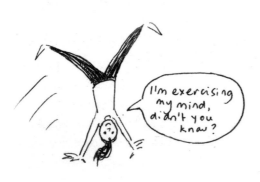

trying to conceive for a while, the stress can take its toll emotionally, and symptoms of anxiety and depression are not unusual. Exercise can often help to manage these symptoms better and maintain mental health, so I wouldn't encourage you to adopt the lifestyle of a couch-potato. As for what form of exercise you should do, my best advice is to **choose something you enjoy, but don't overdo things**.

TIP: **For most women trying to conceive, moderate, regular exercise is best.**

If you've not exercised regularly for a long while and are concerned then do speak to your GP before starting.

3.2i Yoga and Pilates

One of the exercises often recommended to couples trying to conceive is yoga.

'Yoga exercises can help level out a sense of physiological instability by relaxing and gently stretching every muscle, promoting better blood circulation and oxygen supply to cells and tissues which in turn can help to improve the health of the digestive tract, nervous system and other organs. There's evidence to support the notion that yoga can help with fertility issues – not directly, but indirectly – by helping to manage stress,[50] as well as reducing irritability and depression.[51] It can't work miracles – nothing will alter your age or those of your eggs, for instance, so even if you've practised yoga for 20 years, your eggs will still be as old as you are – but can increase energy and improve balance. This can give you back a sense of power and control – and if you're trying to conceive, you might be feeling as if nothing you do can change anything, so I view this as a very positive thing!' **Sarah**

If yoga appeals to you and you've not tried it before, start with a class once or twice a week. Once you learn the basics, perhaps you can carve out some personal time to practise in the comfort of your own home. As soon as you think you might be pregnant, it's advisable to let your yoga instructor know, as they can suggest if and when to switch to a specific yoga pregnancy class, or direct you to pregnancy yoga videos online.

TIP: There are a growing number of fertility yoga practitioners, and a growing number of fertility yoga videos on YouTube for you to follow at home. Find one you like with a voice that soothes rather than irritates you and enjoy some chill-out time.

Alternatively, **you might like to try Pilates,[53] which offers many of the benefits of yoga as it also focuses on developing strength, balance, flexibility, posture and good breathing technique.** However it tends to have much less emphasis on spiritual practices and meditation, which may – or may not – appeal to you.

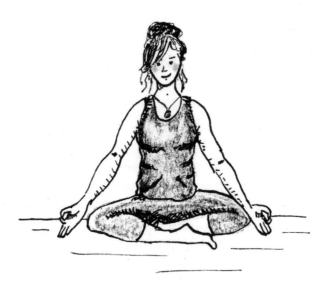

3.2ii Swimming

If you're feeling bloated (a common side-effect of fertility medication and pregnancy), swimming can provide relief as the water supports your weight. It's low impact so doesn't strain the joints either.

> 'Swimming kept me sane when we were trying for our first child; period Day 1 to ovulation I pounded the pool, eating up lengths, initially with anger and frustration that we weren't pregnant, then a desire to be as fit as possible. Post ovulation it was a gentle, calming glide, giving me time to send positive vibes to my growing water baby. It also felt soothingly sociable as I could be with others without having to speak to anyone. Months went by like this and when we did find out we were pregnant, after six rounds of pills to make me ovulate, I had a very healthy pregnancy – and a water birth, of course!' **Paula**

TIP: If you're having assisted conception, most clinics say that swimming is fine whilst stimulating your ovaries or until the insemination but then to stop after your treatment, until given the all clear again.

3.2iii Walking

I love walking – up hills, down dales, walking alone or with friends and family. As well as being a low impact exercise, since learning mindfulness and becoming more aware, even my walk to and from the station and to work is more enjoyable.

TIP: Headspace[54] have some great ideas to incorporate mindfulness into your walking. Any walk, any day, not just weekend adventures can help lift your mood if you notice more, feel more and listen more to yourself and everything around you.

'I sit all day at work and do long days. I knew exercise would help me to manage the stress around trying to get pregnant in a more useful way than a large glass of red, so I got an app for my phone, linked it to my watch and now I count my steps. I've got a few of my weight-watching colleagues in on it and often a few of us will go for a walk at lunch time. It gets quite competitive, and is a good distraction too.' **Claire**

If you prefer walking for a purpose and like canine company, you might like to investigate the *Borrow My Doggy* website.[55] It's a great way to ensure you make a weekly commitment to exercise and you'll have a walking partner who listens intently, is often up for a cuddle and never says the wrong thing!

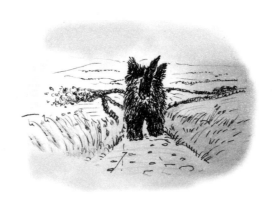

3.3 Alternative therapies

There's not space in this book to examine *all* the alternative ways to prepare your mind and body for conception. You might like to consider:

- Acupuncture
- Herbal remedies
- Homeopathy
- Massage therapy
- Mindfulness
- Reiki
- Traditional Chinese Medicine

...for instance, and we'll look at a few of these here.

3.3i Working with your body

One of the most appealing aspects of alternative approaches such as acupuncture, Traditional Chinese Medicine and massage therapy is that **therapists aim to work *with* your body**. Perhaps it's because many of these disciplines have different cultural origins from western medicine and, broadly speaking, tend to view the mind, body, spirit and emotions as connected. **Holistic medicines[56] thus consider the whole person in the quest for optimal health and wellness.**

> 'With both my acupuncturist and my herbalist, in my initial appointment, we discussed who I was, what I did and what I am normally like when well. Above all, I didn't get medicalized. I didn't get told I was **ill**. I like that approach – to be treated as a whole person. We can have discussions of "I'm in this place in my life..." so I don't feel I'm being told something is wrong, there's no negativity. It's not about "take this pill and the symptoms will go away." It's about supporting me through this difficult, challenging experience.' **Holly**

3.2ii More time

Sarah says, 'There can be another positive aspect to alternative therapy: **one of the things you tend to get – and this is no small thing – is time.'** There's very little alternative therapy that is available for fertility issues on the NHS but at least paying for a private consultation means you tend to get more than ten minutes, which is what a GP is allocated for each patient.

> *'With a reputable alternative practitioner, I find you invariably have an hour as your first appointment. They listen to your story and get the whole picture of your body changes – your symptoms, your emotions, your work, your creativity – all of it.'* **Juliet**

3.3iii Finding a reputable practitioner

So far, so enticing. The problem with alternative therapies is how to sort the wheat from the chaff, or more precisely, the charlatans from the conscientious practitioners. Conventional medicine is controlled by statutory regulation to help ensure that doctors are properly qualified and adhere to certain codes of practice.

Your safest bet is to check that your therapist is registered with an organisation that is itself registered with the Professional Standards Authority[57] – as is the case for anyone listed with the Complementary and Natural Healthcare Council[58] or the British Acupuncture Council.[59] Other professional associations hold membership lists or registers of practitioners of specific complementary and alternative medicines, such as the British Homeopathic Association, The Reiki Association and the UK Register of Chinese Herbal Medicine.

As to whether alternative therapy *works*, I'm aware that to enter into this argument is to open a can of proverbial worms. I can give you my opinion, (and so could Sarah), and as in the next couple of sections have done so, but please be aware that this is subjective. So in addition we've tried to provide links to clinical research where we can. On the whole we'd say that, **if a treatment is improving how you feel either physically, mentally or both, and you can afford it, continue, because your wellbeing is the most important thing of all.**

3.3iv Acupuncture

Acupuncture, an ancient Chinese medicine, involves the usually painless process of placing extremely thin needles into the skin along specific 'acupuncture points'. **Acupuncturists view these points as nodes where lines of bodily energy converge. The needles help to open any blockages** and restore balance to the energy flowing through our bodies, which in turn helps to regulate hormones, increase the blood supply to our (fertility) organs and promote a sense of calm. Usually a series of treatments is needed to get the best results, and the amount suggested is revealed after the first exam and treatment.

Although these lines of energy do not correspond to any actual physical structures known to western medicine and skeptics argue that acupuncture benefits are the result of the placebo effect, having said I wouldn't be subjective, I'll confess, I *love* acupuncture. I've tried it on many occasions – for a whiplash injury to my neck, for frozen shoulder, a knee pain and thumb pain too. I even tried it when trying to conceive naturally to try to make my periods more regular. In each case I felt it worked for me, and there's been the added benefit that I've felt very relaxed afterwards and slept really well.

'I'd been diagnosed with Polycystic Ovarian Syndrome as a teenager; 'Verity'[60] – the support organisation for women with PCOS – recommended acupuncture and it really helped. Later, with traditional medication, my PCOS was well managed, but I had to stop the meds to try to conceive and my system went awry again. Again, here acupuncture really helped. It made a difference physically, but also I felt I was taking myself somewhere to help holistically and I definitely felt emotionally better.' **Flora**

TIP: You can find a specialist acupuncturist with additional training in fertility via the Acupuncture Fertility Network.[61]

When you are trying to conceive naturally, acupuncture can be helpful as it has been shown to be good for relaxation and alleviating stress. Whether it can boost fertility levels remains unproven, however, and there remains no confirmation that acupuncture is effective in increasing the success of assisted conception.

3.3v Chinese Herbal Medicine

In China, the ancient herbal system of medicine still forms a major part of healthcare provision and is made available in state hospitals alongside western medicine. The tradition goes right back to the 3rd century BC, and in its broadest sense Chinese medicine includes herbal therapy, acupuncture, dietary therapy and exercises in breathing and movement (tai chi and qi gong). Some or several of these may be employed in the course of treatment.

Chinese Herbal Medicine, along with the other components of Chinese medicine, is based on the concepts of yin and yang. It aims to understand and treat the many ways in which the fundamental balance and harmony between the two may be undermined and the ways in which a person's Qi or vitality may be depleted or blocked. Specific symptoms such as infertility are believed to reflect an imbalance of Qi, and clinical strategies are based upon diagnosis of these indicators.

'I'm not going to accept a hard, masculine, medicalized style of approach. I prefer a gentler, holistic style of treatment that takes time – that's about rhythms and the cycles of life. After all, that's what we're going through – trying to conceive is the most natural thing in the world. The most important thing is to honour that and look after ourselves. We don't have to be out there striving to sort it instantly – we have to honour the transformation. And what's why I want to go through this naturally.' **Holly**

A key component of Traditional Chinese Medicine is herbs. The herbs prescribed by practitioners are often made into teas which rebalance the energy flow to treat a person holistically, rather than focusing on the symptoms.

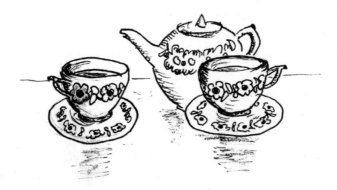

'The tea prescribed for us both tasted so disgusting, I was pleased to switch to a pill format. But even if we'd had to stay with tea, it still would have been worth it, as for us it worked. Having had unsuccessful IVF, with TCM I became pregnant after three months – and this was after we'd been told we'd need to adopt or use donor eggs if we wanted a family. It also really helped Mark to sleep better and boosted his libido.' **Julia**

There is an association of Traditional Chinese Medicine practitioners,[62] but not a specialist fertility division.

Please note: **If you are having or planning assisted conception, it's important to let your consultant know if you're been taking Chinese herbs, they may suggest stopping them as they can impact on the effectiveness of western medication prescribed for your treatment.**

3.3vi Mindfulness

One of the biggest buzzwords in psychotherapeutic circles is 'mindfulness'. Put simply, mindfulness entails focusing your mind on the present moment rather than the past or the future, and in this respect reflects much more ancient Buddhist teachings. Its proponents say that we can spend so much of our time going over the past or worrying about the future that we end up missing much of the richness of the life we have right now. Mindfulness practice offers the opportunity to wake up to our lives in this moment, which can help us to live with greater presence, aliveness, clarity and enjoyment.

Mindfulness meditation, which can be used in conjunction with CBT, has been shown to reduce stress and anxiety and the National Institute for Clinical Excellence (NICE) now recommends mindfulness-based courses for people with recurrent depression.

> 'A few years ago I suffered an episode of severe depression and anxiety. I had a course of Cognitive Behavioural Therapy, and it was then that I discovered mindfulness. I cycle regularly and practice yoga too. Whilst I still get tired if I overdo it, and have the odd weepy day, I am now much better at managing my physical and mental health.' **Vicky**

Like Vicky, **I'm a fan of mindfulness**. This might sound simplistic, but in mindfulness training, I honestly feel that I discovered *me*. **I learned acceptance of the self, and this is only one of the ways mindfulness helped to promote my emotional wellbeing**. Becoming more aware of how I was feeling, learning to be at peace with myself in the moment whatever my situation, helping me to cope better by drawing on strengths I might have otherwise have overlooked in a busy world – it gave me all these tools, too.

Learning to be mindful can be fun; online tutorials, apps, books, videos and podcasts are plentiful.

TIP: One of the most relaxing mindful exercises can be colouring. Sarah's book, *Making Friends with Anxiety: A Calming Colouring Book* includes tips on managing worry and stress alongside black and white illustrations specially designed for you to colour. This can be really helpful for fertility anxiety as there's just you, the book and your pens or pencils.

TIP: There are many mindfulness relaxation visualisations and meditations on YouTube. Find one with a voice that doesn't irritate you and that's not too long. 5-10 minutes is plenty when your head is full of worries about trying to conceive! And don't worry about whether or not it focuses on fertility – in the beginning it's just about learning to be still.

'We found a mindfulness app we both liked so we could listen together when work got too stressful for us both. We thought it was preferable to relationship counselling as we felt that we were fine, but our work life balance wasn't. It really helped, mainly because it gave us time to be together, supporting ourselves and each other, not thinking about anyone or anything else. I carried on using it during my first pregnancy and when we couldn't get pregnant again, it helped me to manage all my NCT friends having their next child.' **Lou**

We will return to the subject of Mindfulness when we get to Chapter 6: 'L' is for Loss, as it's here we'll be looking in more detail at the emotional effects of trying to conceive.

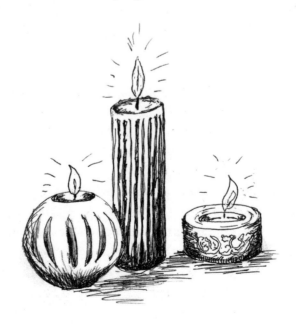

3.3vii Reflexology

Having someone mess with my feet wasn't my idea of heaven, but to ensure I'd tried (almost) everything to boost my own fertility, I had reflexology too. My reflexologist was a former ballet dancer so at least I could feel confident that she'd have seen feet worse than mine!

Reflexology was documented by the Egyptians around 3000BC. It involves using pressure points in the feet, each linked to a specific organ or system in the body, promoting positive energy flow. Specific protocols are followed when treating different fertility issues in men and women, but it can be great for general relaxation too, helping to cope with the emotional impact of trying to conceive. It promotes a sense of calm integration, and can help manage anxiety by reducing the impetus into fight-or-flight mode.

More recently reflexology of the hands and face has enabled people who don't like having their feet touched to benefit. Again individual pressure points are believed to link to different organs or systems within the body.

'I don't know what I expected, tickly feet I suppose, but it was different to how I imagined as I felt things going on in the rest of my body whilst the reflexologist was pressing my feet. Hitherto, my periods had been very clotty and long, sometimes really heavy. After a few sessions, when my next period came it was five days not 15, and I felt healthier during it. That was a while ago, but reflexology is the one treatment I continue to dip into as it gives me a real boost and leaves me feeling energised during the day and sleeping better too.' **Jane**

'My mother-in-law bought us a spa voucher for our wedding anniversary, and she thought we'd have a his-'n'- hers day, but we asked if we could split it so we could have a few reflexology treatments during our treatment cycle. Jason doesn't like needles, and we wanted to have the same treatment even if we didn't do it together. Reflexology was the perfect solution.' **Francesca**

TIP: If the treatment appeals you can find a specialist reflexologist with additional training in fertility issues via the Association of Reproductive Reflexologists.[63]

3.3viii Hypnotherapy

Hypnotherapy is useful if you want help detaching from your conscious, busy life so you can explore what's going on in terms of unhelpful patterns of behaviour.

When someone is 'hypnotized', they enter a very relaxed state, helping them feel much safer, which can heighten their sense of clarity and objectivity. The power of suggestion whilst in a relaxed state makes it easier for individuals to allow changes to be made so they feel better or behave in a more helpful way. Thus hypnotherapy can be effective for helping to manage eating disorders, phobias and insomnia and in helping to boost confidence, especially during exams, tests or first dates. In relation to fertility, hypnotherapy can help overcome fears of anaesthesia, for example, which may prove helpful ahead of tests or treatment.

> *'I loved my fertility hypnosis CD. I thought it was so relaxing, really good at helping me to get to sleep. When our treatment didn't work, John wondered if falling asleep during the CD somehow missed the end bit about pregnancy and stopped some part growing or developing. He apologised, he said he was being silly, but I blame myself that maybe he has a point.'* **Laura**

TIP: There are several hypnotherapy professional bodies, and if you're thinking of trying it, do ask if the individual hypnotherapist has fertility experience or specific fertility hypnotherapy training.

A word of caution about alternative treatments
Laura, like many of my clients, found hypnosis to be really helpful at promoting relaxation during stressful times, but if there was medical evidence of its benefits to promote an increased pregnancy

rate, it would routinely be included with treatment by all fertility clinics. It isn't! The same is true of the other therapies we've explored in this chapter.

In conclusion, Sarah and I agree that if an alternative therapy is helping you to relax, do more of it. Often this may help put you in the mood for sex too, which can only be good news if you're trying to conceive! But if you're not enjoying the therapy and/or are just participating out of a sense of duty, then it's worth trying something else.

Sarah says, 'It's also important to remember that fertility is impacted by age, so I wouldn't advise anyone to spend years and years on alternative therapies if nothing seems to be working. In this instance it's important to investigate assisted conception sooner rather than later.' I agree, so this is the subject we'll look at next.

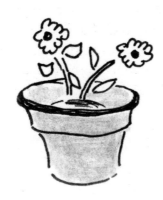

4. 'T' IS FOR TIME TO GET HELP
COMMON REASONS FOR SEEKING ASSISTANCE WITH CONCEPTION, AND WHERE TO GO

Like many women, I spent most of my twenties and early thirties trying not to conceive and assumed that, when I was ready to become a mum, I'd discard the contraceptive pills and bingo – baby! Having moved to a new home, my husband and I were ready to start a family, and marked the occasion by throwing my contraceptive pills on a barbecue. It was January 18 1997, exactly four years after our first date.

As you'll have gathered, we tried and tried and didn't get pregnant. Eventually we began to flag because of the pressure to have regular sex, and this was when we sought help. For many heterosexual couples, seeking help comes after a pregnancy loss, when they are keen to find out how to prevent it happening again.

Next we will look at the many reasons people seek help with conception including pregnancy loss, being single or gay and keen to have a baby, and infertility as a medical condition. We'll also explore whether to go to your GP or a clinic, NHS or private – and the regulations, rules and rating systems.

4.1 Reasons for needing assistance with conception

4.1i Pregnancy Loss

Around a quarter of pregnancies end in loss, and the most common reason is miscarriage.

FACT: A miscarriage is defined as losing a pregnancy before 24 weeks. If a baby is born alive before 24 weeks, even if they only live for a few minutes, the loss is registered as a live birth and neonatal death.

The **Miscarriage Association**[64] notes that the main causes of miscarriage are likely to be:

- **Genetic** – this is when the baby doesn't develop normally right from the start and cannot survive. More than half of all early miscarriages are caused by this.
- **Hormonal** – women with very irregular periods may find it harder to get pregnant. When they do get to conceive, they are more likely to miscarry.
- **Blood clotting issues** – problems in the blood vessels that supply the placenta can lead to miscarriage, especially if the blood clots more than it should.
- **Infection** – minor infections like coughs and colds are not harmful, but very high temperature fevers and some illnesses or infections, such as German measles, may cause miscarriage.
- **Anatomical** – there are three main anatomical causes of miscarriage:
  - **If the cervix (the bottom of the uterus) is weak,** it may start to open as the uterus becomes heavier in later pregnancy and this can cause a miscarriage
  - **If the uterus has an irregular shape**, there may not be enough room for the baby to grow
  - **Large fibroids** are harmless growths in the uterus, which may cause miscarriage in later pregnancy.

From this it's clear that the biggest cause of early pregnancy loss is chromosomal problems that are incompatible with life. So whilst it may seem shocking that one in four pregnancies ends in miscarriage, it's worth reflecting that this statistic is in some sense a reflection of our bodies working *for* us, not against us, even though it may not feel at all like this when you experience a miscarriage yourself.

If the cause of pregnancy loss is identified, a solution to reduce the risk of losing another pregnancy, such as removing a fibroid or prescribing medicine for a blood-clotting problem, will be planned, but often there is no known cause and the general advice is to try again when you're ready. If you are pregnant and fearing pregnancy loss, please do speak to your GP about support.

TIP: This may be upsetting to read and hard to face in the situation, but I feel it's important to say as it is something I wish I'd known myself: if you are one of the many woman affected by miscarriage, retaining the products may make it easier to test what went wrong, and therefore to identify if there is a problem that can be prevented in a future pregnancy. I recommend you contact your early pregnancy unit as soon as you have any symptoms of miscarriage and follow their guidance.

It's also worth emphasizing that there is *no proven link*[65] between miscarriage and stress levels, so if you have a miscarriage, **please don't blame yourself**. If we had the capacity to 'stress ourselves' into not remaining pregnant, by the same logic there would be no need for contraception and no woman would ever experience an unwanted pregnancy. The reasons for successful pregnancy and pregnancy loss are much more complex than that.

TIP: There is lots of support available for pregnancy loss via the NHS and the Miscarriage Association.

The NHS state that most women who have experienced a miscarriage go on to have a healthy pregnancy.[66] Nonetheless, although the loss becomes manageable over time, it's not uncommon for there to be moments when the memory is still painful.

'I didn't realise just how strong I was until I experienced a miscarriage. Possibly it's stubbornness, too, but whatever the reason, I went from being broken, devastated, to trying again for a baby after a couple of months. We went on to have two children (now 11 and eight years old) but every now and again I find myself upset. There's still sadness, and I think about how different life would be if that first pregnancy had worked. We would have a 13-year-old too.' **Jo**

4.1ii Being single and keen to have a baby

There are many reasons why, as a single woman or man, you might decide to go it alone and have a baby. You may be happy on your own and see yourself remaining that way, or you could still be seeking the right person but feel that time is running out biologically so you'd best try conceiving sooner rather than later. Whatever your circumstances, these days it is much more acceptable to choose not to settle for the wrong relationship in which to become a parent, and in my work I've observed a rise in the numbers. When I began supporting people hoping to conceive whilst working with Fertility Network UK back in 2003, I'd only speak with a single woman around every two or three months. By the time I started working as a Fertility Counsellor in 2011, this number had grown noticeably, and now about one in three of my clients is single. Admittedly single men are more of a rarity; most single men I work with these days are planning to co-parent in non-intimate relationships. To date I've only worked with a couple of single dads who wish to remain that way and use a surrogate.

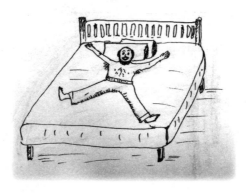

Given it takes two people to conceive,[67] single people will need assistance with conception. Sometimes they do so via home assisted conception services, and many use private clinics, here in the UK anyway, as frustratingly there is very little NHS support available to help in such circumstances.

Donor sperm is readily available for single women hoping to conceive in a clinic, donor eggs and a surrogate can take a little more planning. Reassuringly most clinics will have a patient coordinator who supports parents through each stage of the surrogacy process.

TIP: Going along to a local or national fertility show[68] can give lots of different options around pathways to parenthood for single people.

FACT: If you're in a lesbian relationship and not married or in a civil partnership, the donor is usually considered to be the legal parent of your child.

4.1iii Being gay and keen to have a baby

Lesbian couples may decide to try to conceive at home with assistance from a known donor.

FACT: If you're in a lesbian relationship and not married or in a civil partnership, the donor is usually considered to be the legal parent of your child.

It's important to be aware of the law, and if you're in any doubt, please seek legal advice from a professional.[69]

Lesbian couples also have the option for intra-partner egg-sharing. This is where one woman donates the eggs to the other who is going to carry the pregnancy. If you are planning to conceive this way, treatment must take place in a clinic through In Vitro Fertilization, commonly called IVF.

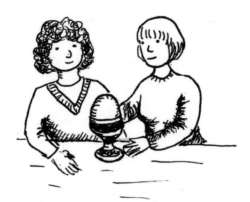

If you're a gay man[70] and want to father a child, you can co-parent either through a home arrangement or via a clinic. If you are co-parenting with a lesbian couple who are married or in a civil partnership, for instance, you may not be the legal parent of your child. Surrogacy is another option for gay couples to have their own child too. If your surrogate is single, then either dad can be named on the birth certificate as the second parent; this is just one of the reasons why the professionals who work in clinics always ask patients to seek legal advice – to make your treatment gives the outcome you want.

Tip: Stonewall[71] produce guides around parenting options and the legalities of parenting for gay couples. Do visit the website for the latest information.

Online sites such as Pride Angel[72] can provide surprisingly easy access to known donors and co-parents. Some are willing to help with home conception, others only via a clinic. If you are trying at home I always suggest having implications counselling, as you would at a clinic in a known donor or co-parenting situation. You can find a specialist counsellor via BICA or the National Fertility Society.

And of course whether you're gay, straight, single, paired up or otherwise, if you are open to alternative pathways to parenthood, adoption is also an option. We'll be returning to this subject in more detail in Chapter 8.

4.1iv Infertility as a medical condition

The World Health Organization[73] defines infertility as:

> 'A disease of the reproductive system defined by the failure to achieve a clinical pregnancy after 12 months or more of regular unprotected sexual intercourse.'

They go on to say that infertility is a disability:

> 'Disability: Infertility generates disability (an impairment of function), and thus access to health care falls under the Convention on the Rights of Persons with Disability.'

4.2 Where to get help and what to expect

If you are experiencing infertility as a heterosexual couple or are trying to conceive as a single person or in a gay relationship, the first port of call is usually your GP.

TIP: Some GPs are more sympathetic and responsive than others, so do ask the receptionist if there's a GP with a specialism or area of interest in fertility at your practice if you're not sure who to see.

4.2i Making friends with your GP

You may well wish to visit your GP as a couple, but most doctors prefer to deal with one patient at a time. They will usually be happy for you both to be in the room together, however, as long as you are both comfortable with the prospect. If so, I recommend you make two individual appointments and both attend the surgery.

Sarah asked her GP friend, Dr Patrick Fitzgerald, who co-authored *Making Friends with the Menopause* to put together some pointers to help you get the most from your appointment. What follows is his advice.

Dr Patrick: It's well worth arming yourself for the consultation with your GP beforehand. Bear in mind **your doctor has 10 minutes to go through your concerns. Still he or she will need to examine you as necessary, formulate a plan you and your GP are both happy with, and then write it up.** Sometimes patients can forget that their doctor is human too, and he or she will be affected by the stories they hear every 10 minutes, and it's good to remember that. I'd suggest that **the following may help you plan for an optimal consultation:**

1. See the right doctor – do you want a male or female? Ask. Do you not want a specific doctor because of previous problems? As Tracey says, ask the receptionist's advice if you're in doubt. It may mean you have to wait a little longer to see the doctor of your choice, but it will be worth it in the long run.

2. Make a list. You're here about your desire to have a baby and possible fertility issues. So write your concerns down – all of them, but stick to the subject. If you start asking about a different issue you're going to flummox the GP who has 10 minutes to try to support you with a highly complex problem and you're not going to get the focus you need. (Have I said 10 minutes enough times?) Make another appointment if you have a second, unrelated problem.

3. Tell the GP what you think may be going on. It helps establish your concerns around your symptoms and you can also be reassured if you are worried about something unnecessarily. However, if you think you may have something more serious then tell the doctor too. e.g. family histories of diseases – these vital clues help to build a picture.

4. Allow the GP to ask you questions, even if they seem irrelevant. NHS.co.uk has details of the questions the doctor is likely to ask you, but please trust that your doctor will be sifting through information[74] to make sure nothing untoward is going on. Smoking and alcohol information are needed –

don't be upset, it's not a judgement or being nosey – we need this to help find the safest way forward.

5. If you're a woman, your GP may weigh you to see if you have a healthy body mass index (BMI). **He or she might ask to examine your pelvic area** to check for infection, lumps or tenderness, which could be a sign of fibroids, ovarian tumours, endometriosis or pelvic inflammatory disease (PID). If your doctor is male and needs to do an internal examination, it's common practice for someone else to be present in the room when he does so.

6. If you're a man, your GP may check your testicles to look for any lumps or deformities and penis to look at its shape and structure, and for any obvious abnormalities.

7. Ask your GP what the options are. After a physical examination, you may be referred to a specialist infertility team at an NHS hospital or fertility clinic for further tests. It may be a referral to a clinic or a specialist. What do you expect to happen? **Tell them what you are expecting.** If your GP doesn't know then they may assume other ways forward.

8. Make a follow up appointment, if needs be, to discuss any test results.

9. If you feel you didn't connect with your GP, don't get angry. It may have been the consultation before yours that involved something so upsetting that they couldn't concentrate. It may be that they should retire! Make an appointment with another doctor until you find the one who suits you. Though be warned: it may not be the one who gives you lots and lots of time as they may be dithering around decisions.

Remember, your doctor is there to support you. They can't fix all your concerns in one appointment, but they will listen to your worries and try to provide guidance to the best of their abilities.

4.2ii Testing your fertility hormones

When I was trying to get pregnant, my GP advised me and my husband to try to conceive naturally, having intercourse every 2-3 days for a year or two. In some parts of the country it's standard for doctors to recommend trying for three years before further checks are requested. But **if you've been trying for six months and haven't conceived, then I always suggest asking your GP to check your gonadotropins and sex hormones as tests can help to identify any problems. It's also a good idea to request a semen analysis.**

TIP: Did you know you don't have to go to your GP to get a referral to a fertility clinic? Self-referral is an option, if you're willing to pay for fertility tests. Often clinics provide a Fertility MOT or Fit For Fertility Package.

Whilst it's always worth checking with your general practice first, especially as **fertility treatment can be expensive and is not covered by medical insurance,** it's distressing to be in limbo when you're desperate for a baby. We weren't aware that we could self-refer to a private clinic, and our GP wasn't very proactive. In fact, we'd been trying for over a year when we got a letter from our clinic saying there was 'only another eight months to wait'. By this point I'd got myself pretty wound up about not getting pregnant, so I called the clinic to ask if there was a cancellation list. It was only then I was told that we could self-refer privately, which we did immediately, and we got an appointment for the very next day. With hindsight, I could have saved myself several months of angst if I'd known this was an option sooner. So if you are keen to speed things along and can afford to, I'd recommend following a similar course.

Medication[75] such as Clomifene[76] (Clomid), which encourages **ovulation, may be prescribed if hormone tests identify a problem, especially if ovulation isn't happening as it should.**

4.2iii Additional fertility tests – for women

If your periods are really heavy or irregular, then your GP may request additional tests or arrange for a referral to a fertility clinic straight away. Here it's likely you may undergo one of the following:

- **Pelvic Ultrasound** – this can be abdominal or, most often, internal and is used to assess the uterine cavity, looking for irregularities such as fibroids.[77] The ultrasonographer will also look at your ovaries, checking the size and the surface for cysts.
- **Hysterosalpingogram (HSG)** – this is a radiologic procedure where a radio-opaque material is injected into the cervical canal in order to investigate the shape of the uterine cavity and the fallopian tubes and an X-ray taken. A normal result shows the filling of the uterine cavity and both fallopian tubes with the injection material spilling out of the ends, confirming they are free flowing and egg can meet sperm. In private medicine, this procedure is called a HyCoSy, the same procedure, but done with a contrast medium that shows up on ultrasound not X-ray.
- **Hysteroscopy**[78] – a small telescope with light and camera is passed through the cervix to enable the radiographer to see the inside of your uterus. If the purpose is investigative, it's unlikely you'll need an anaesthetic. Hysteroscopes are also used in small procedures such as the removal of small fibroids. This is often done under a local anaesthetic.

TIP: If you are having a hysterosalpingogram or hyster-oscopy and there is *not* a plan for any anaesthesia, I always suggest asking if you can take Buscopan, which helps to relieve painful abdominal cramps, ahead of the procedure. They can be painful, especially if you've not given birth.

- **Laparoscopy** is a surgery used to find problems such as cysts, adhesions, fibroids and infection. A thin, lighted tube is put through an incision in the belly and tissue samples can be taken for biopsy through the tube. A laparoscopy is

77

always performed with anaesthesia and can be used to confirm a diagnosis and/or remove fibroids or cysts that might prevent a pregnancy. It can also be used to treat endometriosis,[79] which we mentioned it in Chapter 1.

4.2iv Additional fertility tests – for men

As with female patients, your GP may request additional tests or arrange for a referral to a fertility clinic straight away. Here it's likely you may undergo a semen analysis. **A sperm test checks much more than just the number[80] of sperm that are in each sample.**

- **Volume** – how big the sample is
- **Viscosity** – how watery or claggy the semen is
- **Count** – how many sperm there are
- **Motility** – how well the sperm move
- **Morphology** – what the sperm look like

TIP: Most fertility clinics would prefer you to provide a sample at your appointment, so you don't have to store or transport it. If you're asked to produce a sample it's always best to obtain it after 2-3 days abstinence, by masturbation, as opposed to withdrawing during sex, and all clinics provide a room where clients can masturbate in private for this purpose. The sample you produce should be collected in a container (usually provided by a clinic), so it's sterile and sperm friendly.

4.2v Support with tests

TIP: If you're undergoing tests, it can be helpful to find support from others who understand.

'I found the information on Fertility Network UK[81] very useful. I also spoke to someone on the support line and we arranged to meet

another couple through the forum who were local before we went to the clinic. It was so helpful – I'm not a 'Jilly Joiner' type person usually, but I was so relieved to know it wasn't just me.' **Paula**

If any of the tests performed by your GP do indicate a treatable reason for not getting pregnant, once treated, frustratingly you often have to try again for a year or two before getting a referral to a fertility clinic.

4.2vi NHS or private?

Up to this point, if you live in the UK, it's likely you'll have been able to get your tests on the NHS. But should you need further treatment at this point, it turns into what is often referred to as a 'postcode lottery'.

Whilst the National Institute for Health and Care Excellence, NICE,[82] produces a guideline for the treatment of infertility, there is no obligation by individual Clinical Commissioning Groups (CCGs) to provide a service or, if they do provide one, for it to be in line with the NICE Fertility Guidelines.

TIP: Find out about your regional funding for fertility on the Fertility Fairness[83] website.

Where NHS treatment is available, there may be additional medical or social criteria to the criteria stipulated in the guideline. These include different upper or lower age limits, whether you already have a child or children – in some cases your eligibility may be impacted even your offspring don't live with you and were conceived in a different, earlier relationship.

'Getting treatment for fertility problems on the NHS seems very arbitrary. I can see the relevance of age, but the criteria should be consistent across the UK. Instead it depends where you live and that is grossly unfair.' **Sarah**

TIP: Fertility Fairness provide information, support, and guidance on how to challenge local fertility funding.

'When a colleague suggested I appeal for NHS funding to cover my fertility treatment and write to my MP, I thought there was no way that I'd succeed. But I have found infertility far more distressing than anything else I've been through – including cancer – so I decided to give it a go, and we managed to obtain funding for two IVF cycles. Even though my NHS cycles weren't successful, I think they helped us to plan and decide if saving for more treatment was sensible. The cycles also meant our private consultant had more information so could adapt subsequent treatments accordingly. The NICE Guidelines says three cycles of IVF, because you learn a bit about how you respond and how you cope emotionally each time. I am pleased it worked the third time, our first with our private clinic, as that was definitely our last cycle.' **Fiona**

4.3 Fertility Clinics

Your GP may prescribe medication to promote ovulation, but most tests and fertility treatments take place within a HFEA regulated clinic. Should you not be eligible for NHS funding, you may wish to pursue private healthcare.

4.3i Choosing a clinic - regulations, rules, and ratings

Whilst you may not have spent too much time selecting a clinic hitherto,[84] at this point it really is worth taking a step back to make sure you get the best quality care.

Fertility Network UK[85] produce a factsheet to help you choose a fertility clinic that is right for you. One of their suggestions is to review the patient information, to see the amount of attention given to patient care.

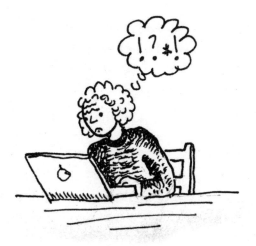

National regulation of all fertility clinics is overseen by the Human Fertilisation & Embryology Authority, HFEA[86]; they produce a Code of Practice[87] for clinics to follow which ensures clinics provide high levels of care to their patients, and when conducting research using human eggs, sperm or embryos.

You can compare your local clinics – both NHS and private – via the HFEA[88] website. The clinic ratings include success rates and patients' views about the treatment they received. Clinics often also have open evenings or events which can be very helpful. They can help you sense if you feel comfortable in the clinic and what the journey there is like for you – whatever treatment you have, it's likely you'll be going many times!

All clinics will do their best to try to provide successful treatment, but some clinics are more willing than others to take on clients with particular problems.

'I've heard that some clinics refuse to treat clients with more tricky medical conditions because they fear their success rates will be negatively impacted. It strikes me that this is unethical.' **Sarah**

TIP: As well as finding a clinic where you feel comfortable, it's vital to get advice from your consultant on your *individual chance of success* before deciding on treatment.

FACT: Success rates shared are representative of the patients seen. They show comparisons by age and treatment type, not the fertility levels or medical conditions of those attending.

In the next chapter we'll look at the different kinds of assisted conception, giving you an overview of the routes most commonly taken, should you decide to have further fertility treatment. It's also worth saying at this point that some people choose not to put themselves through the stress, and that there is nothing wrong with taking this decision. Fertility treatment is emotionally and physically demanding, and you may decide not to pursue it.

> *'I had a history of fibroids and got to my mid-thirties without finding a committed relationship. I decided not to pursue single parenthood – I've respect for those who do, but I was sure I couldn't cope with raising children on my own. I also couldn't face the physical trauma, so assisted conception wasn't for me. I decided to direct my creative energy into writing novels instead.'* **Sarah**

There is never a guarantee that treatment will be successful, so remember, you don't *have* to have any further assistance with conception at all.

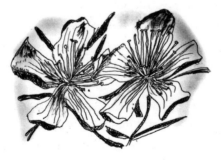

5. 'I' IS FOR IVF
AND OTHER FORMS OF ASSISTED CONCEPTION

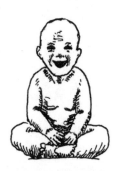

'We're not desperate enough for a child to go through IVF, we would rather adopt if we don't conceive naturally.' This was me and my husband: after trying to conceive for a few months, I even called our local council to enquire about adoption so we could begin to make our Plan B a reality. I was told brusquely to go away, try IVF, then go back if that didn't work. So that's what we did.

Whether you also end up venturing down the IVF road or a different one, it's easy to feel overwhelmed by all the terminology associated with assisted conception. IUI, IVF, ICSI... they sound remarkably similar when you're confronted with them all at once, and consultants, nurses and professionals like me can sometimes forget not everyone knows what they are.[89] Seeing a consultant for the first time often brings up a lot of feelings as it is, and if you're anything like me and my husband back then, you'll feel quite churned up by a mix of hope and fear, self-consciousness and vulnerability, so it's wise to **arm yourself by gaining a basic understanding of the different options before you visit a clinic. Sarah and I have written this chapter together to give a broad overview of the most common different treatments, explaining briefly how they work and when they tend to be recommended.** You can find out more about each of them from Fertility Network UK or the HFEA.[90]

5.1 Fertility Treatment

Once you've chosen a fertility clinic, before you commence treatment you'll almost always be given two secondary care tests which will not routinely have been done by your GP. They are:

- **An Anti Mullerian Hormone (AMH) blood test**, which looks at your egg or ovarian reserve
- **An internal pelvic ultrasound scan.** In addition to checking for fibroids and cysts, the ultrasonographer will be looking at the immature follicles on each ovary. He or she will count them, which provides your Antral Follicle Count (AFC)

Together with your medical history and semen test results, your AMH and AFC will be used by the consultant to work out which treatment option and medication protocol is best suited to you.

Please remember that **unfortunately there is no guaranteed way to make IVF work, so it's important you feel comfortable psychologically with the road you're going down.** Do your own background research and allow yourself time to sit with your emotions before your appointment. Some people prefer to keep things as natural as possible and minimize medication and invasive procedures; others want to use protocols that will maximize the chance of getting pregnant in the shortest possible time span. When you are at the clinic, listen to what your consultant suggests and make the decision that feels right for you.

'I am an Ayurvedic Practitioner,[91] and have witnessed many couples conceive naturally with Ayurvedic protocols, so was initially against the idea of using any form of reproductive technology. My husband has a low sperm count, and although Ayurveda significantly improved the quality of his sperm, the increased quantity didn't increase sufficiently to conceive naturally. So after a lot of soul searching, we finally decided to try IVF with ICSI. We chose a London clinic which offers natural and modified-natural IVF (a minimal drug approach) and after several attempts I got pregnant, and am now blessed with our beautiful daughter.' **Clare**

I couldn't see the point of keeping it natural, when natural hasn't been working! I asked the consultant about other tests and he felt we wouldn't need them. I thought, before we started, I'd go for up to five rounds of IVF, my consultant suggested we take things one step at a time. I'm delighted I didn't respond to the medication as after our first round we agreed it was not going to work for us and moved to egg donation, which worked first time. I'd not planned for or considered donor conception, but my daughter is wonderful.' **Robin**

Initial recommendations are likely to be one of the following:

5.1i Timed Sexual Intercourse

This, as the name suggests, is when you time sexual intercourse to coincide with ovulation, and may be suggested if your scans reveal that you are ovulating earlier or later than predicted. You may have tried this at home already (we had), but whilst over-the-counter ovulation predictor kits are extremely useful, they're not 100% reliable. An internal scan, on the other hand, can provide a much more accurate picture of when a dominant follicle is developing. You can then adjust the timing of sexual intercourse accordingly. If you want to minimize intervention, you can do this within a natural cycle. Alternatively, you might choose to combine it with medication which will lightly stimulate the ovaries to produce one, two or sometimes three follicles. **A clinic is unlikely to let you proceed with more than three follicles, as the chance of a multiple pregnancy is then high.**

5.1ii Intrauterine Insemination (IUI)

IUI is a less invasive procedure that places sperm directly into the uterus. The goal of IUI is to increase the number of sperm that reach the fallopian tubes and thus increase the chance of fertilization. Your consultant may recommend IUI in the following instances:

- If you are in same-sex relationship
- If psychosexual problems such as premature ejaculation make vaginal intercourse difficult
- If there is an issue with cervical mucus
- In cases of mild endometriosis
- If sperm is of low quality (sometimes referred to as having 'poor motility')

You can find the NICE guidelines on its use on their website.[92] If you're having IUI in a clinic, the procedure for the woman is likely to be as follows:

- In a natural cycle ovulation predictor kits may be used to gauge the time of ovulation
- Clinics often include a pelvic ultrasound scan to ensure the timing is optimal
- IUI can also be performed after medication has been provided to help the ovaries produce one, two or sometimes a maximum of three follicles

Meanwhile…

- The male is asked to provide their sample at the clinic
- The sample is prepared i.e. washed and concentrated. The fluid and sperm with poor motility are removed, leaving the fastest sperm

And finally…

- The sperm are placed inside the uterus using a catheter
- There is not usually any anaesthetic, though if needed some clinics can provide a sedative or anaesthetic for the procedure

IUI gives sperm a head start, but still requires it to reach and fertilize the egg on its own. It is a less invasive and less expensive option compared to In Vitro Fertilization, however, so some specialists may suggest, if appropriate, that you try it first.

'I thought IUI would be really painful, but I experienced less discomfort than with a smear test. I'm pleased that I tried it first as I was keen to avoid the stress of IVF. Whilst I know it's only supposed to give the same chance of success as trying naturally through sexual intercourse, I'm single so IUI was preferable, and it worked for me, not once, but twice.' **Ruby**

The importance of counselling

Whilst we're focusing on clinical protocol and procedures in this chapter, throughout your treatment, **I can't underline the value of counselling strongly enough**. Some clinics don't provide routine counselling, others simply offer a one-off appointment or counselling for some treatments and not others. However, **I always suggest meeting with a counsellor, ideally sooner rather than later, so they can support you on your journey through assisted conception**. As you'll discover when you read on, IVF and ICSI are complicated enough, never mind using frozen embryos, a surrogate or donor conception! These circumstances are ethically and emotionally complex and can bring up a lot of feelings concerning our ability to parent, our bodies and how we feel about others involved. We've devoted the next chapter to the subject next – **'L' is for Loss** – but a book can never be a substitute for seeing a counsellor in person, where you can talk and be individually supported.

TIP: You can find an independent specialist fertility counsellor via BICA,[93] but first do ask at your clinic.

5.1iii In Vitro Fertilization (IVF)

IVF is a form of assisted reproductive technology during which the process of fertilizing eggs with sperm is done outside of the human body. The term IVF comes from the Latin 'in vitro' meaning 'in a glass'. Fertilization used to be done in a glass test tube, hence the term 'test tube baby', but now it's common to use a petri dish. The term 'petri dish baby' doesn't have quite the same ring to it though!

IVF is used to treat many causes of infertility including

- Damaged or blocked fallopian tubes
- Severe endometriosis
- Severe male-factor infertility
- Unexplained infertility

As with all reproductive technology, there is not a 'one-size fits all' approach; your treatment plan will be formulated after looking at your test results and past medical history. There are many different drugs that can be used within different protocols, but broadly speaking the three main types of IVF cycle are:

- **Natural or Mild** - your body follows its natural cycle or mild stimulation is used to generate just two or three follicles
- **Flare or Short** – medication is prescribed from Day 1 of your cycle. This enhances the effectiveness of your own hormones to encourage a larger number of follicles to develop on each ovary
- **Long or Down Regulation** – medication is prescribed to 'switch off' your natural hormones, creating an artificial menopause. This allows the medication prescribed to work without any interruption from your own hormones

Eggs are collected when they are mature, but before ovulation.[94] At this point in your cycle they will be loosely attached or no longer attached to the inner wall of the follicle and be moving freely in the follicular fluid. This means they can be removed relatively easily using an ultrasound probe, either under a heavy sedative or general anaesthetic. A very fine needle is then guided to drain each of the follicles. The fluid containing the egg is collected by the consultant and passed to the embryology team.

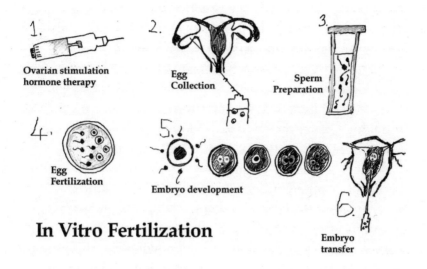

1. Ovarian stimulation hormone therapy

2. Egg Collection

3. Sperm Preparation

4. Egg Fertilization

5. Embryo development

6. Embryo transfer

In Vitro Fertilization

Once checked and prepared, the eggs are left in an incubator with several million sperm surrounding each egg in the hope one sperm will successfully fertilize each egg. The embryologist will check the following morning and call to let you know how many eggs have fertilized, and how many embryos are developing. They may tell you straight away that they have a plan to transfer one or two embryos in a day or two, or to wait and see if they grow on to be a Day Five embryo, called a *blastocyst*.

At the optimal time for each embryo, decided by the embryologist, the embryo is transferred into the uterus. It's usual to have only one embryo transferred at any one time, but after discussing with your consultant they may agree to transfer two. Eggs which are fertilized successfully but not transferred can be frozen to use in a later treatment cycle.

If embryos are to be transferred within the same cycle this is called a *fresh embryo transfer*. It's performed by passing a catheter through the cervix and the embryo is placed within the uterus, guided by ultrasound.

Egg and Embryo Freezing

Egg freezing is carried out to save women from having to undergo repeated cycles of egg collection. It means your eggs will be kept frozen 'in time', so to speak, and is also an option for women who wish to delay trying to conceive.

There are many reasons women may choose to freeze their eggs. Some cancer treatments can impact fertility, for example, so it's a good idea to harvest eggs first. Whilst reproductive technology has come on in leaps and bounds over the last 40 years, there is still little (arguably nothing) that can be done to prevent a woman's eggs from ageing with her. Eggs in younger women tend to have less chromosomal abnormalities, so have the potential to give a greater success of a pregnancy in the future. Against this backdrop, some women choose to freeze their eggs, knowing that there are no guarantees but that it may enable them to use their own eggs to achieve a pregnancy after their natural fertility has declined. However every woman's chance of success is individual, so if you are considering egg freezing, do see a consultant to find out your individual chance of success.

Eggs for freezing are collected as described above, regardless of the reasons. They are then stripped of surrounding cells, assessed for maturity and *vitrified*. Vitrification is a fast-freezing process where the water is removed from an egg, which prevents ice crystals forming as an egg is thawed. (Picture what happens when you take frozen food from your freezer – if you put it on a plate to thaw, after a short time, you'll notice a white crust of ice crystals. Before the advent of vitrification, it was common for ice crystals to cause the fragile egg shell to disintegrate, rendering them inviable. With vitrification, more eggs can survive being frozen and thawed.) If eggs are thawed and fertilized, they can be re-frozen as embryos for future use.

Frozen embryo transfer (FET) is done to enable a further chance of pregnancy if a fresh embryo transfer was unsuccessful, or for a sibling in the future. If embryos have been frozen, they may be transferred on a natural cycle, or medication may be prescribed to help optimise the lining of the uterus ahead of embryo transfer to promote implantation.

Eggs and embryos are frozen at -196°C and can be stored routinely for up to ten years. However if a woman has or is likely to have a medical condition where she is or is likely to experience premature infertility, storage can be extended up to 55 years.[95]

A note about ethics:[96] With many forms of assisted conception there are ethical considerations and for some people and campaign groups the issues involved become highly charged. For the sake of brevity we have not gone into them here, but it's worth being aware of the arguments to make sure you feel comfortable with the route you are taking. The Progress Educational Trust is a good source of information.

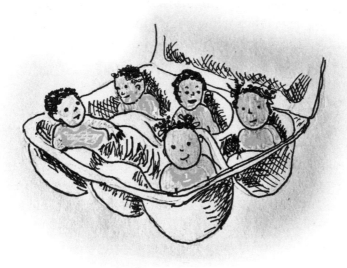

5.1iv Intracytoplasmic sperm injection (ICSI)

If a semen sample contains a small number of sperm or lots of sperm but just a small number with normal shaped heads, then using a microscope to select the best sperm and injecting one sperm directly in to each egg can help to increase fertilization rates, but does not necessarily increase pregnancy rates.

> **FACT: Whether or not to use ICSI may be decided prior to treatment where male factor infertility is identified, or be planned on the day the eggs are collected and the quality of the fresh semen sample is shown to be poorer than was anticipated.**

5.1v Intracytoplasmic morphologically selected sperm injection (IMSI)

Where there appears to be a sperm issue but it's difficult to identify which are the 'best looking', a stronger microscope can be used. The microscope used for ICSI magnifies the sperm 400 times, but for IMSI it's *7000* times. With a microscope that powerful it can be much easier to find the sperm of the highest quality and select them to inject directly in to the egg.

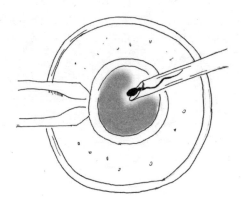

> **FACT:** Selecting the right sperm and injecting it directly into the egg can improve fertilization rates, but does not increase pregnancy rates. This is because a successful outcome is never down to just the egg or just the sperm, it's always both that have to be 'good enough' to achieve a pregnancy.

5.1vi Donor conception as a recipient, a donor or both

Donors enable people without viable eggs and/or sperm to become parents. Donation thus offers hope to many couples and individuals who would not otherwise be able to have children. Some people choose to use a donor they know, such as a friend or a relative.

When looking for a sperm or egg donor some choose to go abroad, but the advantage to using a licensed clinic in the UK is you can be confident of tighter legislation that focusses on the future of any child conceived: you will be able to find out information such as a sperm donor's ethnic group, personal characteristics and so on. Your child will also be able to access this non-identifying information about the donor when they reach 16 and in the UK, the identifying information of the donor at 18.

The commitment of UK donors can come as a surprise to many; egg and sperm donors both attend counselling, have a thorough medical, genetic testing and additional screening; for egg donors, an IVF cycle to get to egg collection, though for sperm donors it's a much longer process. There is often a weekly commitment of around six months to attend the sperm bank or clinic to provide a sample, with a few days of abstinence before each deposit. At the end of the donation programme, the donor has a well-earned break for six months, whilst his sperm remains in quarantine. He then repeats his screening tests and only when all the results are in is the sperm available for selection by recipients.

> **FACT: Only around 2% of sperm donors make it through the donation process.**

The figures are slightly higher for egg donors, who are often more aware of their fertility prior to coming into the clinic to be tested.

It is not uncommon for a woman to donate eggs during her own donor conception treatment. Sometimes she will recognise that she is receiving sperm donated by someone who wanted to help her to become a parent and will 'pay it forward' by donating her eggs to someone else.

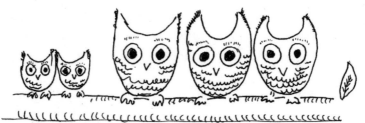

In spite of fears at the time, the removal of anonymity for donors in 2005 did not reduce the number of people donating in the UK. Quite the opposite! The result is that now we have better informed donors at regulated clinics, and egg and sperm banks have invested to recruit and support donors with the same level of care that is provided to patients. Now we have a well-regulated, robust and child-focused system that promotes openness from the beginning for everyone and helps to ensure that the welfare of both donors and recipients is given proper consideration.

This said, **donor conception is not something to be undertaken lightly**. It's worth being aware of is **the HFEA Code of Practices**.

'The law states that, where a woman who has consented to her male or female partner being treated as the legal parent of any child born as a result of her treatment, and the partner has consented to being

the legal parent, treatment may continue after the point at which consent is given only if the woman and her partner: (a) have had a suitable opportunity to receive proper counselling about the implications of treatment in these circumstances, and (b) have been given proper information. When people seek treatment using donor gametes or embryos, they must be given information about: (a) the importance of informing any resulting child, at an early age, that they were conceived using the gametes of a person who is not their parent, and (b) suitable methods of telling the child this.'

It can also come as a surprise to be advised by your consultant that you should inform a child early about being donor-conceived and you may wish to discuss how you feel about it. In the UK counselling to explore the implications of donor conception ahead of donating is usually routine, but some clinics and egg and sperm banks allow you to opt out, and if you're conceiving overseas, it's often not included at all. I feel that this is unfortunate as it can bring up a lot of issues. If a donor sees themselves as a genetic parent, albeit an absent one, there can be lasting implications and sense of loss for the relationship with a child conceived with the egg or sperm they donated – and that's just one example.

There is a growing science called Inter Personal Neuro Biology[97] which reinforces just how important pregnancy is to the developing baby. **It's been shown that the relationships that we form before birth influence how we think and feel in the future.** At all stages of life around 80% of human communication can be non-verbal – we use vocal tones and frequencies, gestures and body language to help us understand our relationships, especially between a parent and child. Which is why it's so important to feel accepting of the decisions around your pathway to parenthood. If a parent conceives through donated sperm, eggs, embryos or uses a surrogate (see 5.1vi below) and sees the donor or the surrogate as an absent genetic parent, why wouldn't a child believe that too? That belief could possibly create a sense of loss, sadness or abandonment for a child, springing from feeling their genetic parent could – or should – have been there for them.[99]

We'll look more closely at the emotional impact of alternative conception in Chapter 6, but if you're offered counselling, I'd urge you to have it.

In addition to counselling, donors and recipients can access specialist support, information and resources via:

- **The Donor Conception Network**[100] – guidance, support and information to families who have used donor conception to conceive
- **The National Gamete Donation Trust**[101] – support and information to egg and sperm donors in addition to information about embryo donation
- There are also **sections on the HFEA website**[102] for donors, parents through donor conception and children conceived through donor conception

---

FACT: These days, donor conception with egg donation is routine in many clinics for women up to the age of 50. This allows us to extend our years of potential for parenthood, as our uterus remains able to grow babies long after our eggs are viable.

5.1vi Surrogacy

Surrogacy is used when a woman is not able to carry a pregnancy, or when a gay man is keen to become a parent, and needs a woman's uterus to carry the child. So it may be that you come to surrogacy having exhausted other forms of assisted conception, or, if you're a gay man, it may be your first port of call. There are two types of surrogacy:

- **Straight** – when a surrogate's eggs are used along with sperm from a male intended parent
- **Host or gestational** – when eggs and sperm come from the intended parents; donor eggs *or* donor sperm may be used,

but not both. At least one intended parent must be a genetic parent for parenthood to be transferred from the surrogate to the parents

> **FACT: Surrogacy is legal in the UK, but advertising for or profiting from surrogacy is not permitted.**

At birth, the surrogate is identified as the legal mother, although if you are conceiving with the help of fertility treatment in a clinic, simplified consent forms enable a more straightforward process for all parties. If your surrogate is single, either intended parent can be nominated as the second parent.

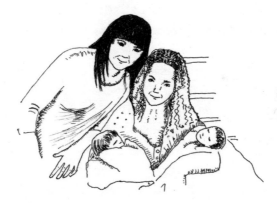

> **FACT: If your surrogate is married or in a civil partnership, her spouse or partner will be identified as the second legal parent. In order to obtain a parental order and become the legal parent(s), at least one of the intended parents must be a genetic parent of the child conceived.**

TIP: If you're considering surrogacy, I always recommend the three main UK surrogacy organisations: Brilliant Beginnings,[103] Surrogacy UK[104] and COTS.[105] They each work slightly differently, but all provide excellent levels of support to both intended parents and surrogates.

5.2 Trying again

Having outlined all these incredible forms of reproductive technology, it's important to remind you again, dear reader, that there is no guarantee your treatment will work. As recently as forty years ago most of these options were not available (the first 'test tube baby' was not born until 1978[106]) and whilst your chances of success might be an awful lot better than when Louise Brown's parents had her, nonetheless, **the majority of women under 35 have per-cycle success rates of approximately 1 in 3[107] with IVF**. As Resolve (the U.S. Infertility Association) puts it: 'Having this perspective may help you think about trying more than one cycle, and feel less discouraged if the first one doesn't work.'[108]

> *'Over a period of six years, I believe I did everything I could to support my body to become pregnant naturally and eventually ended up trying IVF, as my 'last resort approach'. Those years were an emotional rollercoaster, but they taught me that there was something more than just me, my husband and science that makes life happen. There was a third person involved with her own idea of when she wants to come. In the moment that I eventually surrendered control and let go of it all, my daughter arrived. The experience taught me to accept what lies beyond my control, to be flexible and to trust the bigger picture of why this was happening – qualities which help me enormously as I now mother my healthy, happy daughter.'* **Rebecca**

Whatever your personal beliefs when you set out trying to get pregnant, **I don't advocate making a fixed plan because we have no way of knowing how you'll feel next week – let alone next month or year**. Assisted conception is a difficult enough journey, without beating yourself up if you don't stick to the route you mapped out for yourself at the start.

Our IVF didn't work, so we ploughed on with IUI, this time using donor sperm. You may decide to call it a day. Many couples, however, do try again, so next we'll look at four occasions where my clients appear to be consistently harder on themselves when planning more treatment, in the hope that if you're in a similar situation, you can be a little kinder to yourself. The first of this is...

5.2i Trying again after unsuccessful treatment

Negative results from a home pregnancy test, from a blood test at the clinic or urine test with a GP, can all bring a similar initial reaction – numbness. It might be a shock or you might be prepared, but it usually takes a while to process the news. Even if you've had an inkling your treatment hasn't worked, you can feel silly for being surprised. Especially because, as we mentioned in Chapter 2, when the embryo implants, some women experience a discharge or blood spotting.[109] (Even professionals can be misled; those of us who work in clinics all seem to know someone whose period seemed to have started, but whose test came back positive and who went on to have a healthy pregnancy.) This means that until you've had a test confirming your treatment wasn't successful, there is always, sometimes frustratingly, hope.

- **If you have been trying to conceive through timed intercourse or IUI,** your treatment may well have covered more than one cycle anyway. If this is so, a review or follow-up appointment would usually be scheduled after three cycles. You don't have to wait this long however – if you feel it would be helpful, ask for one sooner.
- **A follow-up appointment after an IVF cycle is standard in most clinics** and, if you're a private patient, this is usually included in the cost of your treatment. Some clinics may suggest you have to book your appointment within a certain timeframe if you are planning to go straight into more treatment as tests may need to be repeated or additional tests performed before trying again. This illustrates the hazard of planning perfectly, however, as you might feel you want to discuss what's happened sooner or later than originally mooted.

If you're feeling distressed and would like to talk to someone, counselling for support can be accessed at any time. I always suggest popping in or having a telephone appointment with a counsellor – although it's not possible at all clinics, it's always worth asking, as having a quick chat or check-in can help to promote a robust foundation of support before your next treatment cycle. **You may also like to explore accessing alternative therapies (such as those we looked at in Chapter 3)**. You might choose to continue with treatments you've had that you found helpful, or you might decide to change your approach. These decisions are yours to make and talking the options through can help you feel supported.

When you try again, **your treatment cycle may follow the same protocol as your last one, it may be changed slightly or your consultant may suggest a completely different treatment** – there isn't a set guide. For each individual patient your consultant will look at multiple factors including:

- Scan results from during your treatment to see how you responded to the medication
- How many follicles developed on each ovary and at what speed they grew
- How many mature eggs were collected if you went through an IVF cycle
- How many eggs fertilised and how each embryo developed
- The quality and quantity of sperm that was used

Additional tests or supplements may be recommended, and amendments made to your next treatment plan to give each egg and sperm the best chance.

'I was quite frustrated our consultant wanted me to follow the same routine with the same drugs. The doctor explained that sometimes it's about luck which Jack found really irritating, especially as it costs so much. But we decided to stick with it for one more cycle; I liked the clinic, especially my nurse. We got fewer eggs the second time so

*I'd given up hope, but the doctor was proved right in a way – luck **did** seem to play a part. Not only did it work and we had Freddie, it gave us Lucy from our frozen embryo too.'* **Helene**

TIP: If a plan is prepared by your clinic (and it usually will be), it is worth reminding yourselves that you don't have to start straight away, or even at all.

When we acknowledge we can always stop, we take control around our treatment. You have absolute control whether to continue, stop, wait or explore other options and/or other clinics.

5.2ii Trying again after pregnancy loss

After my miscarriage, I was amazed at how quickly we wanted to get going again – after a chemical pregnancy,[110] where I had a positive pregnancy test, but my period started a few days later, I needed much longer to be ready to try again. Sometimes there's no rhyme or reason why we react differently, and that's how it is for many of my clients. Each loss is different and we can't foresee how we'll feel.

'Initially my partner Clare and I had planned to do three IVF cycles – we were lucky our treatment was on the NHS and the wait was only about six months. Our first cycle went fine – we got pregnant. But our first scan at seven weeks showed there was a foetus with no heartbeat. I had to have a procedure to remove the products of conception[111] and was emotionally numb for a few weeks, but after a normal period, I felt reenergized and wanted to get on with it - we still wanted a family. But the next cycle we miscarried at five weeks and it was awful. I didn't have to go to hospital and so my partner thought I'd be ready again more quickly than before, but I didn't have it in me. We're planning to try again but this time Clare will be the one having treatment.' **Susan**

After miscarriage we begin to heal and grieve for the loss of our wanted child; treatment can re-traumatize us, causing us to re-remember what we've been through. It's quite common for a positive pregnancy test to increase anxiety and a negative test to cause a sense of relief. Anxiety comes from fearing another loss, relief from knowing you don't have to experience it again. **Being kind to yourself, being mindful and accepting feelings as appropriate given all you've been through can help to alleviate the impact**. Seeing the counsellor at your clinic can be really helpful, and I also recommend accessing support through the Miscarriage Association.[112]

5.2iii Secondary infertility

You have one little person, they're wonderful, so you'd like another! Should be simple as you've done it before and your body knows what to do, shouldn't it? Unfortunately, it's often not as easy as this,[113] and around one in seven couples can experience secondary infertility. Whether you conceived naturally or at a clinic, secondary infertility can be as stressful as trying to conceive before having a child, sometimes more so.

> *'Now we have Robbie and he's just perfect, so I thought it would be much easier to try for a second child. For me everything is still perfect, but if we conceive again, that makes it even better. I found it really hard to see Mel struggle so much – it felt like Robbie and I weren't enough. It took counselling for me to see how different it was for each of us, and even with counselling I still found it hard.'* **John**

Support is really important for secondary infertility, because so many people just don't 'get' how difficult it is. Do please share your feelings in the *Making Friends with Your Fertility* Facebook group if you feel able to. Fertility Network UK has a support group just for secondary infertility.[114]

5.2iv Trying again with donor conception

When you've tried to conceive with your own eggs or sperm, making the decision to move to donor conception can be tough. It isn't for everyone, but when we were considering moving over, I found time was important; it's so helpful to have a bit of space to consider if you are comfortable with the implications of your decisions, for you, your family and most importantly any child conceived. Again, counselling beforehand is usually routine, and I'd heartily recommend it.

TIP: I believe comfortableness in donor conception is key to a successful outcome; comfy donors and comfy parents all promoting comfy children growing into comfy adults. If you're not comfortable, I suggest a delay prior to treatment, allowing time for accessing support, seeing a specialist counsellor and meeting other parents. Be kind to yourselves and create the space to breathe until you've enough clarity and the reassurance that donor conception feels right for you.

When you do begin your next cycle, with a child or after loss, with the same treatment plan or a different one, with your own eggs and sperm or those from a donor, you might try not to get too excited. But to your unconscious, you're right back at the start, with the potential for success. So it's back to high-highs and low-lows. Practise self-care and seek support and, if you're reading this with a friend in mind, offer them a quiet, accepting hug and suggest they drop into the *Making Friends with your Fertility* Facebook group.

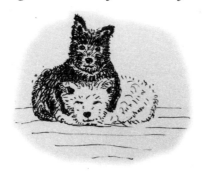

6. 'L' IS FOR LOSS
THE EMOTIONAL IMPACT OF FERTILITY TREATMENT

In Chapter 1, we acknowledged that hormones can affect us emotionally. Remember how I said that some women seem blessed with hormones that synchronise, like a ballet troupe, whereas mine are more like a group of toddlers inclined to tread on one another's toes? One example of hormones having an effect on mood is pre-menstrual tension – along with physical symptoms such as bloating and breast pain, many women experience mood swings and irritability in the run up to their monthly period. (While we're on the subject, if you're a sufferer and if the over-the-counter remedies aren't helping, I suggest speaking with your GP and finding out more from the National Association for Pre-Menstrual Syndrome.[115]) Another example is when we go through the menopause, though most of you, dear readers, won't be at that point yet.

If we have fertility treatment, our hormones will be impacted too, but when we're trying to conceive, there's a much bigger aspect of ourselves that comes into play – *our unconscious.* Put simply, the unconscious mind means treatment can bring up 'stuff' for us. (By 'stuff', I mean our individual life experiences, not just facts. Fantasy is important too when thinking about fertility – I'll come back to this presently.) Unfortunately there's no over-the-counter remedy for the unconscious mind and, coupled with hormonal fluctuations, this potent mix can result in emotions that are so intense that often we can feel overwhelmed, occasionally out of control. Certainly I experienced bigger highs and lows during treatment than at any other time. If that sounds an exaggeration, then I'm guessing you're not a reader who has been through fertility treatment, as I'm confident many of those who have would agree that it's not just an emotional rollercoaster – it's like the most extreme theme park ride you can imagine.

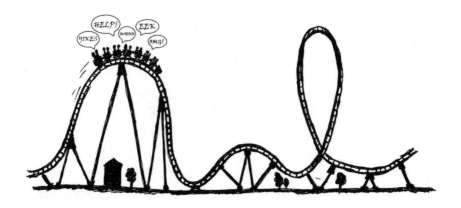

For everyone who's tried to conceive and hasn't (yet), loss is a big part of our situation. How we cope can often depend, to an extent, on what we've had to deal with thus far in life, what we've processed consciously and how things have been stored in our unconscious. One positive effect of past experience is that it can make us *resilient*;[116] sometimes present situations can be *triggers*[117] that remind us of the past in a more negative way. When we look at the loss of a fantasy child we'd envisaged, one that was maybe conceived in a certain way with a special person, born at a point in time we'd planned for, with holidays or work plans amended, just in case... then we can begin to comprehend how important it is to acknowledge fertility-related loss.

In this chapter we'll look at the emotional effect of trying to conceive when things don't work straight away. My hope is that if we understand more about what's going on emotionally, we can take the pressure off a little. We'll quieten the inner critic that says we're failing, and we'll stop berating ourselves as much for not feeling how we think we 'should' feel. **Sarah says, 'Learning how to manage and be "friends" with the more difficult and troublesome parts of ourselves can be hugely helpful. Our feelings about fertility are very complex, and bound up tightly with how we see ourselves. But if you can find a way through to "making friends" with your fertility, even when you're experiencing problems with conception, that may enable you to be kinder to yourself and more accepting of what does - or doesn't - happen.'**

We will look at:

- **Nurturing capacity** – understanding emptiness
- **Fantasy Loss Ownership** - going with the 'FLO'
- **Understanding the lows** – trauma and loss
- **Understanding the highs** – hope and excitement
- **Forget CBT, let's talk DBT**

6.1 Nurturing Capacity – Understanding Emptiness

I'm blessed that my husband, like good wine and cheese, has got even better with age and still, many years after our own treatment, I wonder what his very own 'mini me' would have looked like. Sometimes it still triggers an emptiness around what might have been, thankfully now wholly manageable, but it hasn't always felt that way.

Not everyone will experience an emptiness when trying to conceive, but daily I work with people who do. Over the years I've developed my own theory, let's call it *The Egg of Emptiness* model, created as I wanted a way to explore the feelings and impact of fertility-related emptiness with my clients.

Imagine that we each have an unconscious nurturing capacity containing our desires to cherish, encourage, develop and protect. I find it helps to picture this capacity as a chocolate Easter egg, with a solid outer shell, and each nurturing activity a chocolate inside. Every chocolate has a different satisfying centre, filling up the egg and contributing to a sense of fulfilment.

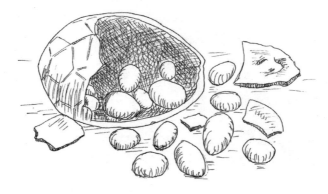

Our nurturing capacity is the same size whether we are single or in a relationship. If we are single, it tends to take a higher number of nurturing activities for us to feel fulfilled – imagine lots and lots of small chocolates in the egg – or sometimes there's a mix of higher value nurturing activities mixed in too – in which case you'd have a few larger chocolates along with several small ones. Our nurturing activities might be walking in nature for instance, or spending time with close friends and family, work too, as we tend to be there a lot. If we are in a relationship (and our partner is worth keeping hold of), then some things in our lives tend to need to give a little, reduce in size or be left behind as there's not enough room to have a fulfilling relationship, together with all our other activities too. (Sarah has pointed out that perhaps this is why some people are inclined to 'dump' their friends when they meet a new partner, and I agree, but we haven't got the space to explore that here.)

A good relationship is like a great big chocolate – and along with a few other chocolates, much of the time it is enough for us to remain fulfilled. However, when we're trying to conceive, we develop an emptiness within our nurturing capacity as we make room to welcome a child. None of us can foresee how much nurturing our

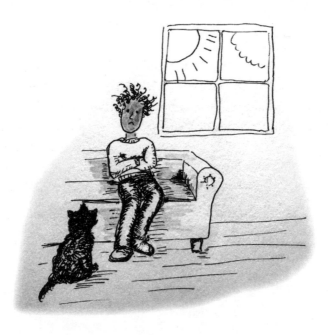

own little person will take, so imagine the chocolate egg shells are parted, but now no amount of chocolates can fill the gap that has opened in between; it's never full up, so we're left feeling unfulfilled. It's like a huge, bottomless pit. We can sometimes try to do more, work harder, see more people, take a holiday, but it can still feel hollow. 'What's the point?' we end up asking ourselves, or 'My mojo left me,' as one client of mine put it.

If we *do* have a child, then we join back together and again feel fulfilled; picture a bigger egg than before, with an extra-large, extra-yummy new chocolate inside. If we *don't* get pregnant and instead embrace a new nurturing plan, be it adoption, donor conception or self-nurturing and not parenting, then we join back together, but that void of potential stays within us. I envisage it is as a Christmas bauble inside the Easter egg, ever so sparkly but ever so fragile, most often safely wrapped deep inside. Mostly, we're virtually unaware of it as our lives become busy and we feel fulfilled in other areas, but every now and again, that bauble feels a bit near the surface as if we may crush it, or it may crush us. But mainly it's manageable.

'I decided if I couldn't have a baby I would find a new job. I did but I still didn't feel happy. I had a great relationship and many single friends thinking I should be grateful for that, and I was… but it wasn't enough.' **Julia**

Feeling empty isn't a *bad* thing: it means we really want a child and have emotionally made room ready to welcome one… or more.
Emptiness is appropriate if you're experiencing secondary infertility too. Secondary infertility doesn't mean that parents aren't grateful for what they've got; to me, it's just a sign that they love their family and there's a void within their nurturing capacity, just about the right size for one more little person. With one child, people tend to understand the desire for a second, but they tend to be less sympathetic if you have three or four and would still like more. Yet if you've the emotional space, of course the desire to fill it will be there.

6.2 Fantasy Loss Ownership – going with the 'FLO'

People who didn't get how I felt when we were doing everything possible to conceive, who wanted to be helpful (you know, the annoying sort), would often say 'Oh Tracey, just go with the flow.' They meant well, but it was about as useful as a chocolate teapot. So I dreamt it up – seriously, I *did* dream it! – my own, alternative sort of flow, 'FLO', which stands for *Fantasy Loss Ownership*.

I have used *change curves* for years. In my life before fertility treatment, I worked as part of a team of occupational psychologists and we used them to help explain how people process change in different stages. They are also often used by HR departments when explaining the emotional impact of redundancy.

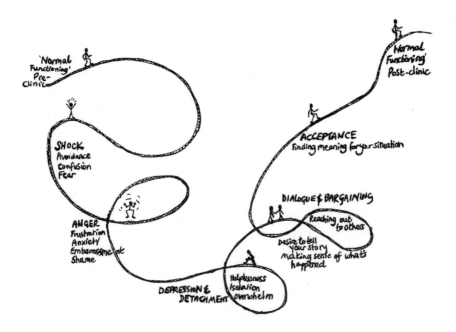

The illustration here shows the different emotional stages, also sometimes called *the stages of grief*, around a piece of string. The string reflects the way that life has many strands, so we often feel all over the place, not neatly intertwined. Equally our emotions are not in any way fixed. We each go up, down, twist, turn and loop back and forth in our own unique fashion. I've used *pre-clinic* and *post-clinic* as the beginning and end of the string here, but it works in many situations and timeframes. We'll look at it here with respect to ourselves as individuals, and in the next chapter with respect to relationships.

In a perfect world, if we're in a heterosexual relationship and want to have a child, it would be conceived during beautiful love making. Whilst rubbish sex with the right person isn't as ideal, for the majority of straight couples, it's still better than needing assistance. **So for those who have been trying to conceive for some time, walking into a fertility clinic – never mind the treatment itself – means that we have to relinquish this fantasy and can trigger a sense of loss**. I've observed that my heterosexual clients in relationships often vocalise feelings such as 'life is unfair' and a sense of anger and frustration, along with the highs of excitement and optimism that they are 'doing something' and there is hope.

For same-sex couples and single women, in a fantasy, conception would probably take place without the need for a donor. Yet they too have dreamed of having a child, often for a long time, and in many cases have saved money as well. This additional planning can create an even stronger belief around how we think we 'should' be feeling, making us even more self-critical.

EXAMPLE

Putting FLO into practice, let's imagine you've been out for dinner to a fantastic restaurant. The food has been exceptional, the service great and the ambience convivial. It's all been so good that while you're there, you book to return again, next time with friends. But when you go back, the restaurant is there, but it's completely different. Instead it's a pop-up venue with a new team taking over each month. How would you feel? In all likelihood it would be a mix of:

- **Shock and confusion** – 'what's this?', 'we weren't told', 'it's not what I expected' – along with fear as you've no control over the situation

- **Anger – 'this isn't fair!' – and anxiety too,** 'what do we do?' Then you realize you're exposed; others know, you invited friends, you might feel shame and embarrassment
- **Helplessness, overwhelm and disappointment**. Or perhaps you'd become detached so the whole situation feels a bit surreal, like watching yourself in a movie... Much safer!
- **You might try dialogue and bargaining** – have a chat inside your own head – 'shall we go, or stay?' or talk to one another. There's non-verbal communication too, when you'll use your senses and gut instinct to assess body language
- **Acceptance,** decision made!

All of this would happen in a matter of seconds – minutes at most. With redundancy the feelings are much more intense and prolonged, so, depending on the individual circumstances, it can several weeks, even months to reach acceptance. Often people are asked to leave very quickly, before anger arrives, to prevent 'a scene'. More sophisticated HR departments might support an employee through the process so he or she can leave at a time of acceptance.

'When our first round of IVF didn't work, I felt like I was grieving, but we hadn't lost anything tangible. Tracey helped to explain that how I was feeling was normal. I've got the diagram on the inside of my cup cupboard door in the kitchen and it reminds me and my husband, that it's OK to be down.' **Jill**

6.3 Understanding the lows: trauma and loss

I view infertility as *wanting to be pregnant and not being*, so it's not limited to those in heterosexual relationships. **Most often in life, our conscious thoughts are in control, but sometimes they are interrupted by our unconscious sending messages which can cause conflicts, leading us to feel anxious or depressed.** Cognitive Behavioural Therapy (CBT) is one type of counselling that can sometimes be useful to help manage these conflicts, and in many circumstances can help us to feel better. However, I've found this approach doesn't tend to work when we're experiencing infertility as it's one time when our unconscious is a bit too big and powerful to respond to our attempts to change how we're consciously thinking. I'll come back to this shortly.

The national fertility charity, Fertility Network UK[118], did a survey in 2016 to coincide with National Fertility Awareness Week[119] (#NFAW), and it revealed that over 40% of women experiencing infertility had experienced suicidal thoughts. To some people these figures might seem alarming, causing them to fear that feeling suicidal is almost inevitable. But to me as a fertility counsellor, they're not surprising: if we didn't have an unconscious all-encompassing urge to have a baby when we're trying to conceive, many women, including me, would settle for a puppy or a kitten from the off, and stop continuing to try!

> 'When learning to manage my own depression better, I found it really helpful to recognise that suicidal thoughts – like all thoughts – can pass. Just as you don't feel the same today as you did yesterday, so you might not feel suicidal tomorrow.' **Sarah**

Infertility is a traumatic time. When we talk of trauma, we tend to think of a potentially life-changing situation over which we have no control. We have no control over getting pregnant, even if we're trying really hard or having fertility treatment. And pregnancy and having a baby isn't just life *changing*, it's life *creating* too.

TIP: It's OK to feel traumatized by infertility. Specialist counsellors[120] have additional training to ensure that appropriate support is available.

Consciously we are very aware we are much more than baby growers. But, when it comes to fertility, the unconscious is in the driving seat of that particular fairground ride.

For women when we're not focusing on our fertility, our unconscious archetypal image of a woman might be a *domestic goddess*, a *sexual being* or a *career woman*. Usually our notion of womanhood encompasses all these archetypes and more[121] – *the witch* is another, more ancient, feminine archetype for instance, *the queen* another. If we're psychologically 'well', these archetypes won't impact unhelpfully on our daily lives, but I've observed that when we focus on our fertility, there seems to be a change in the basic assumptions within our unconscious; the archetypal woman image becomes very primal and *The Earth Mother/ Mother Earth* rises to the fore. After all, our unconscious says forcefully, *'it's why we're here'*. Validation – a confirmation of purpose for human females – is becoming a *Mother*, and if we are not a mother, then we are nothing. For some men the desire to become a father is very much the same, for others the focus is more on *Family*. **Our lows can become very low indeed as we see ourselves as barren, worthless failures.** When we understand the lows are there because we want a baby and have no control, we can relinquish trying to 'get a grip' or 'pull ourselves together'. We can forgive ourselves for not being able to 'think positively' or even 'relax'. Instead, if we try a little self-compassion, we can seek nurturing from someone who cares, who can give us a hug, or listen without interjecting with judgmental advice. **If we are mindful,[122] we can passage safely through the lows.**

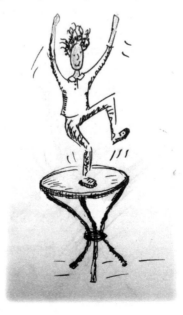

6.4 Understanding the highs

It's not all negative! Knowing we want a baby and are trying, when we are doing something proactive towards conception – for example taking medication or managing our weight to get to a healthy BMI – we can experience huge, unconscious-driven highs. The highs become as high as we can ever imagine: we embody fertile abundance, success and self-worth.

The highs can feel scarier than the lows as it can feel we have further to fall.

For women in lesbian relationships all this can have an added dimension. People often assume as two women you can support each other better. Somehow fertility treatment is easier, it's believed. Not at all! My non-birthing-mum clients – through surrogacy in addition to those in lesbian relationships – often have the potential to be even *more* self-critical. They tell themselves they 'should' understand more and be able to remain calm, zen-like and optimistic. Phooey!

> 'It didn't make sense to me, I felt so positive, like **really** positive, confident I was going to get a positive result on my pregnancy test, but at the same time I felt really scared that even if it did work, it would go wrong. Then in a second I felt lower than I'd ever felt, like someone had turned the lights out and left me. Seeing this illustrated as a piece of string with loads of threads helped to sort the picture in my mind. The string of my unconscious isn't as neatly twirled as in the diagram, though, not in my case.' **Susan**

6.5 Forget CBT, let's talk DBT!

CBT[123] can be very useful in teaching people to identify unhelpful thoughts. It can enable people to develop skills to challenge these thoughts, which can help us change how we think and in turn improve how we feel, and at the same time recognise repeated patterns of behaviour so we can stop making the same mistakes and, hopefully, stay feeling better for longer. I don't really think we should 'forget CBT' – it's great for situations when our conscious thinking is in charge, and it was the main sort of counselling I used when working in a GP's surgery when helping people with moderate depression or anxiety, but fertility is not one of those situations – the unconscious is very much in charge, as I said earlier.

Instead, there's a therapy called *Dialectical Behavioural Therapy (DBT)*[124] that is like CBT but doesn't involve challenging unhelpful thoughts. It was invented to help people with more significant mental health conditions, including Bipolar and Borderline Personality Disorder, where medication alone isn't working. It teaches a person about their condition, educating on how to develop a 'wise mind' to acknowledge big thoughts and feelings that are part of the condition. Then, by creating a toolbox of coping strategies (known as *distress tolerance techniques*) – one of which is mindfulness – it enables better management by allowing the person with the condition to sit with the big thoughts. At the same time it encourages *acceptance*. It's a structured therapy (and in that way is like CBT), but I have found that the principles work brilliantly for anyone finding it difficult to conceive.

TIP: Mindfulness is a useful technique for managing extreme emotions. It helps us to acknowledge exactly how we're feeling *in the present moment*. You can find out more about Mindfulness from the NHS[125], your fertility counsellor or you could ask your GP – they may know about local classes or groups too.

> '*I found the FLO diagram really helpful. Every time I was down, my mum and Andy, my husband, would try to encourage me to be more positive. I felt like I was failing them as I couldn't muster the positive state they wanted. Then, if I got hopeful and was very excited, they'd tell me to calm down and to not get carried away. I couldn't win! The strategies I had in my CBT counselling for depression helped to identify how I was thinking, but sometimes I felt I was letting myself down as I couldn't snap out of it. It was like being in a pressure cooker.*' **Julia**

- If we're down, we beat ourselves up, or someone who cares gives advice telling us we 'should be more positive', 'should just relax' or 'shouldn't be negative'.
- If we're up, we beat ourselves down, or someone who cares gives advice telling us we 'shouldn't get carried away', 'shouldn't tempt fate' or ' not to get too excited'.

We then end up constantly exhausted, as if we're ready to burst, when all we're doing is trying to stay calm.

Instead if we remember 'FLO' and go with the flow, if we're up, we enjoy it! If we're down, we seek support, and remember the lows are appropriate – a reminder of how much we want to conceive and how we are doing something about it.

We can see in the FLO diagram that anxiety and depression are appropriate reactions to exploring our fertility, whether we are trying to conceive now or considering it and planning ahead. Sarah's books *Making Friends with Anxiety* and *Making Friends with Depression* can both be helpful in providing strategies for coping with fertility-related highs and lows. She draws on the tools of Mindfulness Behavioural Cognitive Therapy which is a very similar approach to the one outlined here.

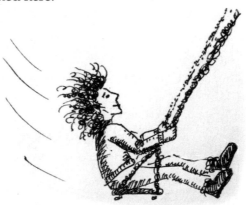

7. 'I' IS FOR INVOLVING OTHERS
RELATIONSHIPS WITH OTHER PEOPLE

Most of us have many relationships with other people, so this chapter isn't just about intimate sexual relationships. In different ways and at different times, our fertility can impact on our relationships with friends, family and at work too.

In this chapter we will look at:

- Fantasy Loss Ownership - FLO in relationships
- Hedgehogs – becoming prickle aware
- Coping with other people's pregnancies
- Sharing information… or not

But first, a word about cake.

Meeting your soul mate is like being given an amazing cake. It's beautiful to look at, expertly baked and tastes delicious. If you're both ready to become parents together, oh my goodness - that cake gets *even* better. It has icing on top, cream inside, it's wonderful!

If you have a child, then a cherry is added to the top. *Bliss.*

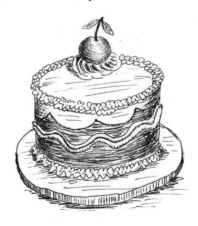

If we don't have a child, or whilst we're trying, a man or non-carrying mum in a lesbian relationship still has cake with icing and cream. It's great – it's just taking longer to get to the cherry. But for a woman trying to conceive, the unconscious may well be saying: 'What's the point of cake without a cherry?' After all, if we didn't have that added drive – the desire to have a child – we'd all stop trying and be content with our cake as it is, devoid of a cherry.

I'm exaggerating here to make a point. I'm not suggesting that *all* men or non-carrying mums feel so relaxed about conceiving, and *all* women trying to conceive so bereft, but my clinical experience has revealed that it's likely their reactions will differ. And with secondary infertility, whilst one has a blissful cherry-topped, cream-filled, perfect cake, with room for another cherry. For the woman trying to conceive: 'What's the point of a cake with only one cherry?' We can feel we're leaving one cherry all lonely and sad by not acquiring a second, or third.

It's important to recognise these differences. **When we understand that although we are in the same situation, we are often thinking and feeling differently, we can see that our strength is in providing support by being available and listening. This is much more helpful than offering support which tries to change or fix the other person, which rarely – if ever – works!**

7.1 Fantasy Loss Ownership - FLO in relationships

We looked at FLO in Chapter 6, so if you've jumped straight into this chapter because you're trying to be more understanding with your partner, daughter, friend or manager it might be helpful to read that one first. (Off you go!)

So, having read about FLO, cast your mind back to an occasion when you shared important news with someone you love and care for and probably respect, when within a few moments it became all about *them*.

EXAMPLE

When I let my mother-in-law, who I am very close to, know we'd need to have donor sperm as a back-up for our first IVF cycle, she said, almost without drawing breath, 'We've had an awful day too. A heron has eaten all the fish in the pond!'

I was speechless.

My mother-in-law isn't usually selfish, self-centred and narcissistic, although I'm afraid I did describe her that way to my husband when blowing off steam at the time. Far from it. She's much more often inclined to be generous and kind – as is reflected by the fact she's happy for me to include this anecdote. But what happens is that we often become like she did when someone shares significant news. We do this as it often acts as a trigger for our own stuff. I know I've done it too.

For my mother-in-law, her shock was that there might be an issue with her son and she believed that I was suggesting it was *her* fault, although what came out of her mouth was something very different.

If we look at the FLO diagram again, this time in the context of sharing our news with others, so we tell them at the beginning and they accept it at

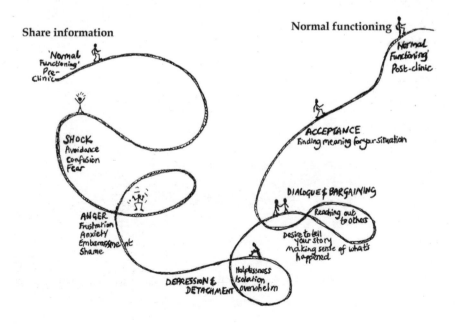

the end, we'll see their responses can also be represented by a piece of string. They are very fluid. Some emotions will be felt sharply, others may be less intense and more manageable.

My mother-in-law's initial shock was quickly followed by shame and embarrassment. After sharing her news about the fish, she didn't call for a few days. I recognise, now, that this was *detachment*; but what she actually said, a bit later, was that she didn't believe we should be so open; she wouldn't be as explicit with any of her friends and she'd appreciate us not mentioning it again. Once again I was left reeling. Sadly, she never reached the point of acceptance as our treatment was not successful – I'm sure she would have come round, though, not least as 11 months later, she accepted the news that we would be adopting with equanimity.

> *'I told a few friends about us needing IVF, and that I was going to share my eggs to help someone else have a baby at the same time. One couple thought it was amazing, but others said they could not do that and my mum was concerned I'd miss my "other babies". I think she was confused, thinking I'd be getting a surrogate to grow me a spare! But once everyone had a few days, most were very positive.'* **Clare**

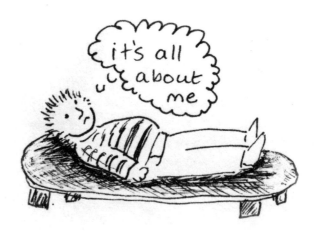

Whatever their role in our lives, **if we have a bit more understanding about what might be going on for the people we**

care about, then we can begin to develop our own what I sometimes call 'an invisible shield of resilience'. With our shield in place, other people's comments bounce off, and don't affect us negatively. My son has a different, more hi-tech safeguard (he's a millennial kid after all) – invisible headphones that mute insignificant chatter. Sarah has a picket fence, as she's drawn below. However we arm ourselves against other people's 'stuff', the important thing is to learn to separate ourselves from other people. Psychologists and psychotherapists often refer to this as being aware of our *boundaries*. **Having strong boundaries can help protect us against feeling battered by other people's negative reactions.**

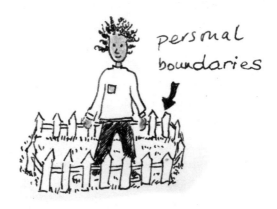

personal boundaries

We can't change how other people process our news, our decisions, or our hopes, but we absolutely *can* control how much we let their process impact on us.

'I was so pleased I'd attended counselling before talking about infertility to my friends. We know a couple who absolutely don't want children, and I've never questioned why, but when I said we were having IVF, the husband was really off with me, then they went quiet. Later, they got in touch as if nothing had happened and I was upset, but Rob reminded me of the FLO diagram and that it was probably more about them than us. Sure enough, eventually it emerged that the husband was anti fertility treatment, and his wife had convinced herself to be positive about not having kids as she wanted to stay with him.' **Fran**

When sharing fertility relevant news, remember to have your virtual shield in place as the initial process will be about them. Stand back, watch the stages, and don't judge too quickly.

I hope these examples show that the people who are closer to us usually process our news with more depth, i.e. bigger feelings and more intense reactions, over a longer time. Meanwhile people we don't know like a new hairdresser or casual acquaintance often seem to take 'our stuff' in their stride.

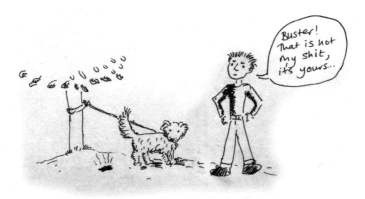

No depth of relationship = no FLO process

This doesn't mean strangers are more supportive, though it may seem that way. It means they have less invested in their relationship with you and so can be more objective.

'It's very easy to get caught up in other people's issues, especially if we're naturally empathetic. No one lives in a vacuum, nor would we want to, but if we're anxious – which I understand is very common when you're having treatment – it can be especially hard to see what's going on as your thoughts are likely to be muddled anyway. Sometimes you can pick up on other people's negativity and this can have an impact on your state of mind too. If you feel your friend or family member is dragging you down, I'd say that it's important to remember to look after yourself first and foremost. If that means choosing your confidantes carefully, selecting only those you feel sure will be supportive, then so be it.' **Sarah**

7.2 Hedgehogs: becoming prickle aware

When thinking about intimate relationships, especially when working with couples experiencing infertility, I often use hedgehogs as a metaphor for us as human beings. The reason? Hedgehogs have soft, furry tummies and backs covered with sharp prickles, so they are both vulnerable and defensive all at the same time.

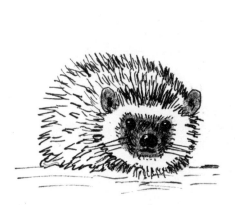
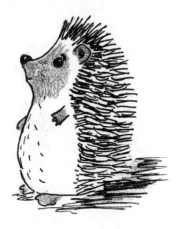

When a couple aren't focused on fertility, I picture them as hedgehogs striding hand in hand along a country path, a path through life; the foundation of which is as strong as the depth and breadth of their relationship. As they move forwards, any obstacle in the way is dealt with. They either climb over or find an alternative route, but the relationship endures. And if the relationship ends and there is a parting of ways, then they continue on two separate journeys, but when we're thinking about fertility, we recognise the lack of control can leave us feeling unstable. For our hedgehog couple this means their stability goes too, so let's move them from the familiarity of their path to a beach. There they struggle with sand, which causes wobbliness underfoot, and unexpected dips and hillocks. Beaches are unfamiliar territory for hedgehogs, and the tools our couple have developed to help them ride out bumpy times are designed for country paths; they don't work so well on a beach. So the unbalanced hedgehog does what hedgehogs do best and curls up into a ball.

When we're having treatment, in addition to feeling physically off kilter and emotionally wobbly just like our hedgehogs, we often invite a whole clinic full of people into a vulnerable part of our relationship. To put it bluntly: this messes with our heads. (We're back to FLO again.) The chance of success can feel amazing or depressing (regardless of what it actually is); one minute we can feel we're absolutely certain to succeed, the next we're convinced nothing will work. And we do what humans do rather well too; we curl up into balls.

If you *both* curl into balls at the same time, then communication stops. More often, one tries extra hard: 'Open up, I'm here for you',

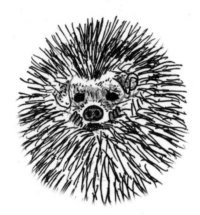

'You can talk to me, it will be fine.' The more one half of a couple tries, the more their soft vulnerable bits get prickled by their partner. And hedgehogs can't hear so well when they are tightly curled, so the closer one gets, the more one presses, the more the one trying to help gets prickled.

We can feel the prickles:

- **Underfoot, as we consider oh-so carefully what to say:** 'I can't say that or they'll take it the wrong way'
- **As prickly anxiety, in the chest:** 'I shouldn't be feeling like this' or 'I should be able to help'
- **As tears pricking behind our eyes:** 'I am often on the verge of crying'

Prickles are a sign that we need reassurance. If you can accept that it's OK to feel however you are feeling, and explain that you just need a hug, a non-sexual massage, a listening ear or words of acceptance, then you can educate those who are close to you to show support, and neither of you should get prickled in the process.

TIP: Hugs can work best when neither hedgehog is curled up. Skin-on-skin contact is healing and reparative, it signifies acceptance of our vulnerable selves and one another.

7.3 Coping with other people's pregnancies

When you're trying to conceive, pregnant women seem everywhere. It's as if every other woman is pregnant. I know this isn't true, but it's how I felt when we *weren't* getting pregnant. I was able to be genuinely pleased when the people at my support group conceived; they so deserved it, but my colleagues, friends and family members who managed to get pregnant and/or became parents whilst we were trying reminded me constantly of what we were missing. I'd even go as far to say I felt persecuted. I recall that I once said someone had 'only got pregnant to spite me'. I don't feel that way now, obviously, but I'm not embarrassed or ashamed by these comments as that was how I felt at the time, and FLO reinforces it's OK to have these thoughts. Reflecting back I can also see how harsh some of my thoughts were and recognise how difficult it was for those close to me, but I think it's important to be honest about just how powerful those thoughts can be.

Our reactions can be confusing not just for those who love us but for us, personally too, especially if we're OK with one woman's pregnancy but not another's; we might cope with a baby shower today, but one we've helped to organise for months is, come the day, an impossible task. When we remember we're not stuck and rigid but we are flexible and fluid, like string or a stream, it allows us to see how we're feeling minute by minute and try not to pressurise ourselves if something feels much too difficult.

127

TIP: Give yourself some time and allow yourself to think and feel however you want – this is the key to coping with other people's pregnancies.

Returning to our hedgehog metaphor, when someone loves or cares for us they might think it's helpful for us not to know about a pregnancy, as we might curl up and get 'prickly' about the news. If we then discover they knew and we didn't, however, we might curl up and get prickly twice. In either case, it's OK. Curling up and being prickly is what we do when we're vulnerable and need to protect ourselves.

TIP: Sometimes it makes things much easier if we can speak to our close friends and family and ask them to let us know privately about any pregnancies, so that we can be spared being part of a grand announcement.

I can also recommend choosing to turn off notifications on social media from people who are likely to share photos of scans, new born babies and so on. Also, remind yourself that if you feel overwhelmed by a situation such as a christening or toddler's birthday you can leave, though it can be easier to have shared with the hosts that you really want to attend, but might have to leave early.

> *'I went to a Fertility Network UK support group when the theme was about other people's pregnancies. I didn't learn a solution, but just talking made it loads easier as everyone there got what the problem was. I don't feel so alone with it now.'* **Jackie**

7.4 Sharing information... or not

Who to tell, what to say, when to say... there's no right or wrong answer. Fertility treatment has no guaranteed outcome, so sometimes people decide to say nothing other than to one another, though that seems rare these days. In some families or cultures there can be a stigma around not having children, for some people talking about fertility feels just too private to want to share, but with one in six couples[126] experiencing infertility, in fact it isn't uncommon at all, and if you tell no one or very few people, it can feel very isolating.

I have mentioned a few times about not being stuck, and that how we feel changes, often. If you tell those close to you, all will process in their own way. Some will be wonderfully supportive, some might back off, and some might ask too many questions or want to be too involved. How they respond will shift, just as your feelings shift too.

'The first time we tried everyone knew, I figured we're a female couple, they'll know we've used a donor so let's be open from the off. But when it didn't work I had to mop their tears. Last time we told no one and that wasn't right either as we only had each other or sometimes we both wished there was someone else to talk to. If we adopt, as this will be our last go, then everyone will know, so we're thinking of being open again, but more for planning if it doesn't work than because that's best for us.' **Jo**

It's OK to tell people you're trying to get pregnant and it's also OK to say you're not sharing details.

TIP: Forums, including our Facebook group can be great, and Fertility Network UK[127] list all support groups in the UK and will support you in setting up your own. However, meeting others in person who are undergoing treatment can be really helpful, whether you have friends and family who know about your situation, or not.

The one thing I do always suggest being open about with the people who love and care for you is donor conception; being comfy with your decisions is what gets modelled to others, and they take their lead from you.

TIP: If you're not comfy with the decisions about your treatment, or not comfy in not having treatment, seek support from a specialist counsellor.

And when thinking about support, your number one friend is *you*, and when we're kinder to ourselves we can begin to let others in to support us too. Sharing with others can help you to help yourself, and as you proceed on your journey do remember the *Making Friends with your Fertility* Facebook group is also there for each step you take.

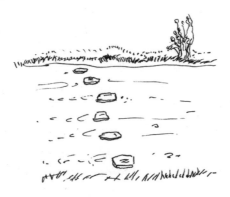

8. 'T' IS FOR THROWING IN THE TOWEL
TIME TO STOP TRYING TO CONCEIVE

Before I got to the point when we stopped trying to conceive, I imagined that ending treatment without a take-home baby would leave me defeated, feeling like a loser. But in the event, it wasn't like that; it was more a gradual shift in our viewpoint, like a pendulum slowly swinging over. The same is true for most people who decide to stop. It's more about reaching a point where it feels 51% OK to find a new plan than it is about suddenly arriving at 100% certainty.

In this chapter we'll look at choices, how and when we choose to stop assisted conception. There are no rights or wrongs about when this might be – it could be after a dozen tries with IVF, it could be before we've had any treatment. We'll also look briefly at some of the possible next steps including adoption and fostering.

8.1 Calling it a day with assisted conception

If there was a perfect time to end treatment that minimised stress, ensured you both felt the same way and provided clarity that there would be no regrets in the future, then life would be much simpler for many of us.

8.1i The financial factor

Whereas couples who can conceive naturally might worry whether or not they can afford to have a child, or a second child, the financial issues are often much more complicated for those with fertility issues. If NHS funding for treatment is available, making the decision to stop can feel much more personal than practical, which is as it should be. But for those who are having treatment privately, having to decide how many cycles you can afford is often a major factor in ceasing treatment.

'Money makes the world go around,' so the song goes, and certainly it's one aspect of private fertility treatment than can cause conflicts.

'We set a figure of how much we'd spend on treatment before considering other options, but we spent that on the first cycle! Instead of stopping, we felt we needed to do one more round and my parents and Sue's mum helped financially, which was really nice, but in some ways brought added pressure – I felt we were letting them down when it didn't work again. We didn't want to continue but our parents insisted they wanted us to be happy and would willingly pay – it felt as much because they wanted a grandchild as about us. So we took some time out then went again, but Sue didn't respond to the medication, so the treatment was abandoned. I'm still in two minds, part of me wishes we'd not gone ahead as it definitely felt we did it for our parents not us, the other part is pleased we did as it gave us clarity that it was right to stop.' **Pete**

Money can cause conflicts not only with other people but internally too. Internal conflicts can be more difficult than those with other people, so finance is every bit as much of an issue for single people as it is for couples.

TIP: There is no right amount of money to spend. Setting a budget can be essential for some and helpful for others but a few people may find it actively unhelpful. However, what is pretty much universally helpful is *talking about it*. The ostrich approach isn't one I'd recommend!

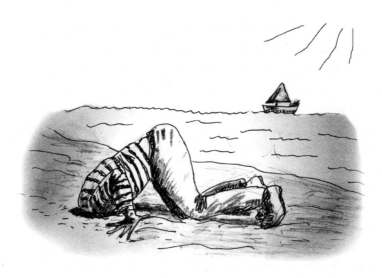

8.1ii The emotional-wellbeing factor

'I know we could have had three cycles of treatment through the NHS, but after two miscarriages, I couldn't even make it to first base. My doctor thought I'd regret not having IVF, but Rob and I knew we were ready to be a family of two – just me and him. Our counsellor helped us to see that if we have regrets in the future, we can look back and know that we explored every aspect of having IVF at the time and we just couldn't get comfy with it. It's the right decision for us not to have treatment. If, in the future, we think about adoption that is another matter.' **Pippa**

Pippa isn't alone in thinking IVF, or any form of assisted conception, is too difficult an undertaking. It's definitely not for everyone, but if you're in two minds about how to go forward then counselling around having – or not having – treatment should be available through the clinic which you considered using.

'The media makes IVF look so great, so simple. "You can't carry one baby? Don't fret – IVF will give you two!" I felt like a moaning teacher, trying to educate those who should be supporting me.' **Pippa**

TIP: When you're ready to stop treatment, the people who love and care for you can take longer to accept your decision, especially if they think you'd make lovely parents. Remember FLO and to give them time to adjust to the new reality.

8.1iii The size-of-family factor

Whilst we often end assisted conception treatment with a smaller family than was hoped for, this is not true in every case...

'I couldn't believe it when I saw our first scan. We only wanted one child, but our first cycle of IVF – with only one embryo transferred – there they were: identical twins. Our cycle had been physically and emotionally tough but once I was pregnant, I loved every minute. We definitely didn't want more than two, though. Our boys were born a little early and we decided that was us done with treatment. But we had eleven embryos in the freezer. Every year we'd get an invoice which acted as a nudge to consider what we wanted to do, and every year I would send a cheque but avoid telling John, not sure if I was more scared of him thinking I was mad for keeping them or if he'd be spurred into suggesting we try again. It was John who realized that we needed to sort it – we'd written our will, and it brought up the issue. We went to see the counsellor at the suggestion of the lab when I called them. This was very helpful – and I came to see I didn't just want them thrown away. I wondered if I should donate them to help another couple, but a family history of breast cancer ruled that out. John was relieved at this; he'd been ambivalent as the embryos were genetically identical to our boys. But he thought there might be other ways they could be useful, so he asked about research. And that's what we did. Our hope is the research they are used for helps other people in the future. Now I just wish I'd not waited nine years before deciding to take action!' **Josie**

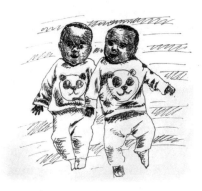

TIP: Counselling support should be available after treatment, and using it to help decide what to do with frozen eggs, sperm or embryos can be very helpful.

8.2 Coming to terms with not having your own child and looking at other options

8.2i Closure with your clinic

When we looked at the emotional impact of treatment, we recognised that it is often traumatic. It's therefore important to acknowledge how important our relationships frequently become with those treating us – the nurses and doctors, ultra-sonographers, phlebotomists, counsellors, and receptionists too.

TIP: Ending treatment also means ending those relationships. Having a closure visit, a follow-up appointment and/or sending a card can all help you to take control of your ending.

8.2ii Acceptance of both positive and negative emotions

Sarah asked what made us decide it was time to 'throw in the towel' and it reminded me what happened. At that point we'd actively got a plan: after numerous tests we were going to have another cycle of

IVF with donor sperm. But when a couple called Dawn and Paul, who we'd known since our first support group meeting over a year before, attended a meeting of the group at our house one evening, everything changed. Dawn said, 'This will be our last group, we've done lots of research and we've decided that we are going to adopt. We've chosen an adoption agency we like and we start the preparation workshops at the weekend.'

The rest of the evening passed in a blur, but I can recall that we grilled them on their research and the agency they'd chosen, keen to find out why they felt it was so right for them, given it wasn't their local council.

At 4am the following morning, we called the adoption agency and left a message requesting an information pack. It was as if Dawn and Paul had given us permission to change our plan – if our friends could do it, so could we! So to answer a question I'm sometimes asked: 'Do you ever come to terms with not having your own child?' I'd answer: 'Yes, or rather we had come to terms with it enough to have talked about not continuing. We'd physically, emotionally, financially reached the point where it felt at least 51% right to stop.' **In other words, we were ready to embrace a different life than the one we hoped for.**

You'll recall that in Chapter 6 we looked at the emotional impact of infertility being unconscious rather than conscious and I mentioned how the classic CBT model isn't particularly helpful in this instance. The same is true when it comes to deciding when to stop trying to have a baby: I don't believe that challenging unhelpful thoughts in an attempt to feel better is beneficial. Instead, acceptance is key.

TIP: Acceptance that *any* thought, *any* feeling is OK is what's important. We don't need to battle positive or negative thoughts. The time it takes to come to terms with not having our own child is not fixed and cannot be rushed.

Situations described as being like an 'emotional rollercoaster' is one of Sarah's bug bears ('My husband pointed out it's become a cliché as it's used as a metaphor for everything from emotions to the economy,' she says.) Nonetheless the phrase *does* sum up this time. There are highs – positive thoughts such as no more juggling appointments, no more injections, no more bloating or scans, especially the ones when you're on your period. But we can feel guilty, sad or bad for being positive, and there are negatives too. Sad thoughts are entirely appropriate; we grieve for the loss of a child that we were ready to welcome, we'd prepared and planned for their conception, and we may have thought further ahead, especially if we'd had donor conception, considering their childhood and the implications of our decisions through to our offspring's adulthood.

We can just start to feel better when a friend announces a pregnancy, or we spot a bump or *baby-on-board* badge and it brings it all back again.

> *'I was numb for about six months, I only realised I'd been numb when I wasn't any more. I'd got up each day, gone to work on the right days, slept well at night, even had sex, for fun. But it wasn't **me**; I think I'd detached too much as it hurt so much. I wanted to stop, but the positive thinking stuff made me feel worse. I "should" be able to cope, nothing had changed, we had each other, no one died etc etc. What I think I wanted was a funeral or memorial service for my embryos.'* **Jacqui**

Self-care is important. When **we accept however we're feeling, we allow ourselves to heal, over time**.

> *'Acceptance is what lies behind the **Making Friends** ethos; it entails being willing to turn towards our experiences and emotions – both good and bad – so that we make friends with them. Whereas if we view difficult experiences and emotions as the enemy, then we end up wanting to make them go away as quickly as possible.'* **Sarah**

Hopefully things will get easier and if not, or your mood seems low for a prolonged period, then please do remember that specialist counselling support[128] is available and well worth seeking out.

TIP: Coming to terms with not having your own child can be isolating. Fertility Network[129] have support, advice and information in addition to their helpline and volunteers. *Saying Goodbye*[130] **hold services for people who have experienced pregnancy loss or the loss of a child and there are a growing number of non-religious services such as** *Give Sorrow Words*[131] **for people who have experienced unsuccessful fertility treatment.**

For each of us the experience of stopping and mourning of loss will be different, so try to listen to yourself and your needs rather than trying to fit your emotions into an imaginary timetable.

> *'I don't know what I did to decide I was ready to look at other options, but I recall that the counsellor at the clinic said "Parenting through giving birth is only one nurturing option, there are others". I think I was closed to other paths to parenthood before, but shortly after she said this, I saw an ad for fostering on the back of a bus and it made me smile.'* **Clare**

We will look at adoption, fostering and not having children presently, but there are opportunities for nurturing which can promote your self-esteem and self-confidence whilst enabling you to support others too:

- Mentoring[132]
- Buddying[133]
- Befriending[134]
- Volunteering[135]

None are guaranteed to make you feel better, faster, however, so it's still important to take whatever time you need to heal.

Letting friends and family know you're taking some time out of thinking about what your future family might look like can give you a break from their supportive questioning.

8.2iii Coming to terms with not having grandchildren

I am mentioning this for two reasons:

1. I hope some parents of people trying to conceive are reading to understand more, to support their son or daughter and I want you to know it's OK to be sad for yourselves about the loss of fantasy grandchildren.
2. Although you might come to terms with not having grandchildren, it does come back, again and again. Sometimes it is more manageable when you have support from friends and sometimes you might benefit from more structured support.

TIP: Specialist fertility counsellors[136] provide counselling for childlessness in addition to fertility treatment and can work with anyone experiencing fertility-related issues. This includes supporting the parents of people adjusting to being involuntarily childless or who have decided to live child-free.

8.3 Adoption

'You can always adopt…' This is the oft-said comment we hear from well-meaning people who want to say something, but remember the unconscious motivation is frequently so *they* feel better. I've observed that many people see adoption through rose-tinted glasses, as if it's a wholly positive solution to childlessness.

*'It was so exciting, we'd seen a perfect little girl in **Children Who Wait**, a magazine from Adoption UK that's like an Argos catalogue of children waiting for a new family. The little girl's social worker and his manager were coming to meet us, and I'd bought new bowls, a new table cloth, made soup and my own bread – Nigella eat your heart out! – I was set to impress. They came, and we thought it went well, but as they were leaving they mentioned that they had four*

other families to see. We were gutted when they went with someone else, and it was like losing a baby all over again.' **Jo**

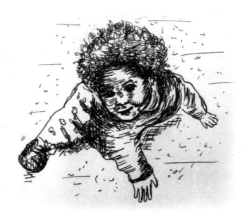

Children needing homes matched with *homes needing children* – sounds simple, doesn't it? But it isn't as straightforward as this so **it is important not to rush, and to take the time to understand the process and the complexities of adoption before being matched with a child. First4Adoption acts as the gateway to adoption information and their informative website details the steps to be taken during the adoption process.**

TIP: If you're keen to learn more about adoption, request a First4Adoption[137] information pack and go along to a couple of adoption information events or open evenings, many of which are advertised on the First4Adoption website.

Alternatively, The Inter Country Adoption Centre[138] provides information for anyone who might want to adopt from overseas.

Everyone who wishes to become a parent through adoption has to be checked out in terms of suitability. So whether you're planning to adopt a child from the UK or overseas, you'll have to be assessed. If you are adopting from overseas you pay for your assessment and adoption administration (and it's often very expensive), but for UK adopters it is free of charge.

For some, the assessment process can feel a bit intrusive; looking into medical history, needing to meet with significant former partners, asking about finances, your relationship, including your sex life and how you've come to terms with not having your own children. If it feels too much, then take time out to consider if it's right for you. Often your social worker, who works with you from assessment through to you becoming the legal parents, will pause the process if he or she thinks that it's too much for you.

If it sounds harsh, like a lot more hurdles to get over, let me explain more. You know how traumatic infertility can feel, what a potentially life-changing situation it is, over which we have no control? It's similar with adoption, but *the person experiencing this trauma is a child*. Any child being adopted will have experienced the distress of separation from their birth family, along with specific and invariably painful circumstances that will mean they need a new forever family. Adopted children often re-process early loss and trauma again and again during their childhood. **The assessment process helps to make sure you understand and can love, empathise with and support your child, without them re-traumatising you.** I'm sure you can see, dear reader, that if a social worker can find a sore spot, or something that feels uncomfortable, it's more than likely an adoptive child would be even *better* at pushing those buttons!

A social worker's job is to optimise the outcome for any child in need. They will ensure that:

- You can provide a robust, stable home
- You are able to meet the physical and emotional needs of a child placed with you
- Your hopes and expectations around working and providing for your family in the future are workable, e.g. you have the ability to take time off when a child is placed
- Your lifestyle and the capacity in terms of time you are able to give to a child are compatible with the child
- Your medical history doesn't preclude your being chosen – if you've experienced depression, for example, and

141

sought support or treatment, it can actually be seen as a strength as it indicates you can ask for help and work through things. Equally a previous cancer diagnosis would not exclude you from adoption, but responsible agencies would seek guidance from your oncologist and doctors to promote longevity of family life to avoid further losses for a child

Just as the welfare of the unborn child is at the heart of regulated fertility treatment, safeguarding and optimising outcomes for children is at the heart of adoption regulation.

It is routine in adoption nowadays for there to be some contact between adopted children and their birth family. Often this is by letters sent on a regular basis with the post-adoption team facilitating a letterbox service. Contact between siblings placed with different families may also be by letter or it might be arranged formally at a children's centre or informally between families.

Meeting with other families early on who are also planning adoption, and speaking to other adoptive parents can be really helpful, giving insight into the realities of adoption and the local support and after care available. And remember, **you don't have to adopt via your local council, so do check out local agencies too.**

TIP: Adoption UK[139] have regional and national events and volunteers often organise local groups or evening social events.

Adoption can be very testing, and children who have experienced a lot of trauma may be too much for you to feel you can cope with.

Adoption isn't right for everyone. If you explore it as an option and it's not for you, don't view it as a sign of your inadequacy; view it as a good thing that you were able to have clarity before taking things further.

If you do decide to go forward, I wish you all the best. My son is 19 now, having joined our family when he was four years old. He's still as cute as he ever was, but these days he's old enough for a pint!

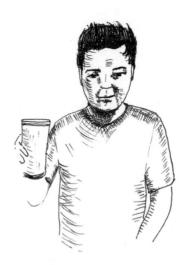

8.4 Fostering

Rexhausting! That was my made-up word to describe our experience of fostering – being as it was rewarding and exhausting at the same time. When we explored fostering in 2014, it was very much as if we were the only foster carers who had adopted previously; most were the other way round, going from fostering to adoption. Others were couples who had had children the 'fun way' and liked parenting so much that they decided to carry on caring for children who needed fostering. There is definitely more of a mix in the past couple of years, with fostering very much presented as something anyone can do. This said, **I'd underline that it is definitely different to parenting.**

Regular meetings with social workers, teachers and birth parents can all be a routine part of fostering, but what surprised us was not so much that, but the length of time it took to sort the basics. Getting a school sorted with just a day or two of notice often means home education for a time, for example, so perhaps it's beginning to be clear why for most types of fostering one of you does need to be available full time. If you're single, it's unlikely you'll be able to manage another job.

There are different sorts of foster carers, specialising in different age ranges of children entering placement, different medical/special needs and different durations:

- **Emergency** – a child's first stop when taken into care. Often a child is placed with little or no notice, so it's usual that experienced foster carers provide short-term emergency care
- **Short-term** – if it is thought that a child will return home or have alternative family carers, then a short-term placement of anything from a night to a few months may be sought. If a placement looks like it will continue, a child will be moved to long-term fostering
- **Long-term** – long-term foster carers provide a permanent home where it is not possible for a child to return home
- **Respite or Short break** – often regular respite or short break fostering is used to provide support within a long-term placement to give the foster carers a break whilst not changing a routine for the child

Joining the Fostering Network[140] can give lots of practical advice, information and support as you explore different fostering options. As with adoption, you can foster through your local authority or with an agency.

Fostering is much more of a vocational profession than adopting in that all foster carers are self-employed and get paid by the local authority or private agency. Thankfully there's a simplified taxation process[141] for foster carers too.

'Being a teacher put me off adoption. I knew I could love other people's children but didn't want to be a working mum, and I'd have had to carry on working if we adopted in order to earn a living. That felt wrong to me: I felt that a child who wasn't living with their birth family would need someone around all the time. Fostering felt right for us both. It took about five months to be approved and Sean came to school and volunteered one day a week to get more hands-on experience with children. It really helped him to see the value in what we were doing.' **Rachael**

It's important to be aware that fostering after infertility can feel very difficult. I've heard people say, 'I couldn't hand them back, it would be too hard' and 'you love them and lose them, what's the point?' But I always say, 'Have a look, find out more, even if only so that you can discount it.'

When exploring adoption, an adoption agency's job is very much to put you off, they want to make sure you can cope with conflict; **but fostering is often well-supported and provides opportunities to build lasting, impactful and rewarding relationships that are nurturing for you and any child placed**. It's often exhausting too, but do find out more about the realities, rather than assume it's not for you. Who knows? You might be surprised!

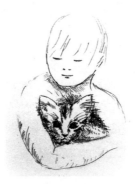

8.5 Being childfree vs childless

'The term "child-free" is used most often to refer to people who have made a choice not to try to conceive or have a child by another way. I guess this describes me, although it makes it sound as if I made an active plan not to do so, which isn't the case at all. For me it just sort of happened, or unfolded, rather than being a conscious decision. I had a deep-seated sense that I did not wish to have a child if I didn't meet the right man from as far back as I can remember, and as I didn't meet that person within the right timeframe, I've never had children of my own. I arrived in this place partly because I loved having a dad as well as a mum when I was growing up, and partly because I didn't feel that I had the mental stamina to do it solo. Yet whilst I'd have liked to have my own children, I can see that this is

very different than if I'd gone through fertility treatment and then arrived at the same decision. I mourn the loss, but I haven't experienced the same level of trauma.' **Sarah**

If you've tried to conceive or have opened the potential to welcoming a child, then my experience suggests that people who focus *only* on the positives of not having children often find the emotions around being childless more difficult to manage. As we touched on earlier in this chapter, being psychically healthy often involves 'making friends' with the dark as well as the light, and acknowledging and accepting loss as part of who you are – something we'll return to in our final chapter. But accepting childlessness *doesn't* mean you can't be positive about the life you have without children. Far from it!

> *'Lying in bed at noon with a glass of fizz, we're having our first official Christmas celebrating being a family of two, celebrating us! We're no longer battling infertility, we don't have to face any more losses. We can have sex when we want it and quality time together. I'm even glad we're seeing our nieces today and friends with children for New Year.'* **Rose**

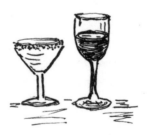

Not having children still carries some stigma and can result in judgement from others, arguably particularly for heterosexual couples, where raising a family still seems more 'the norm'. Being childfree can also promote envy at the life you're able to lead without the demands of children. Having support from others who don't have children can help to ensure you have a space to share the frustrations that these prejudices can cause.

TIP: Support[142] for involuntary childlessness is available. There are many online forums, groups, events and workshops, and of course you can get support from the *Making Friends with your Fertility* Facebook group.

TIP: There is online support for people choosing to live childfree[143] available, and we'd welcome you in our Facebook group too.

> *'When we were trying and people asked how many children we had, I'd avoid answering or change the subject, in the hope people would shut up. Now we've stopped I've got fed up with people assuming my work and our holidays are more important than a family. I'm quite open about the fact it's sad we don't have any kids and I tell everyone I meet aged 32+ to freeze their eggs or try for a baby NOW!'*
> **Jan**

You'll know what feels OK for you, or 51% OK, at least. And talking of endings, for me, this feels the right time to end the journey we've shared in this book. Writing it has helped me make firmer friends with my own fertility, and I hope I have shared some suggestions that can help you to become friends with yours too. Sarah is going to be with you for Chapter 9, 'You'; reflecting on the things we've explored together and introducing a few examples of people who are in the process of making friends with their fertility too.

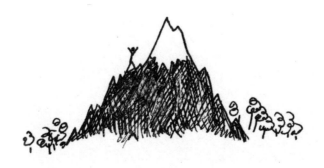

9. 'Y' IS FOR YOU
FINDING YOUR OWN WAY THROUGH

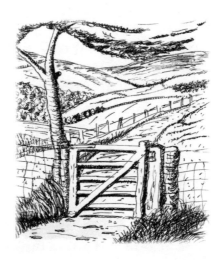

As Tracey says, we're nearing the end of our journey together, dear readers. We've travelled from F, the facts about fertility, through E.R.T.I.L.I. and T, to arrive at Y. But before we go, let's try to get a sense of the entire lived, felt experience of fertility. What follows are the experiences of ten individuals, all with different insights to share about fertility and their feelings on having – or not having – their own children. In one or two of these stories you may hear echoes of what you've been through, or what you might envisage for yourself in the future, which might cause you to reflect upon what 'making friends with your fertility' means for you personally.

'There's no right or wrong way to make this journey. It's about finding your own route through and however that is, it being OK.' **Helen**

Over to you…

9.1 Your stories

9.1i Joanne, 14, who turns to her dad for support

We had learnt about periods in school, but it still felt crazy having to ask my dad for tampons, as Mum's not with us any longer. Dad coped brilliantly, he'd read all about it, even bought books! When I feel rubbish he makes hot chocolate and knows to keep a box in the bathroom topped up with tampons and sanitary towels – he said, 'Every now and again you might need more than a tampon'. He has become an expert. I didn't think there was a problem, but sometimes there seems to be loads of blood and I'm pleased for the extra reassurance I won't leak at school.

9.1ii Chris, who is also 14 and going through puberty

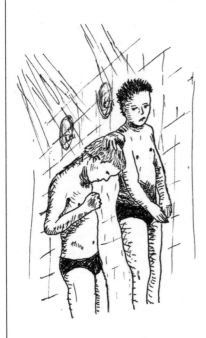

Showers are awful, especially once you've got pubes – it's a nightmare making sure you never look down! No one tells you this in primary school where you just lark about and can laugh about who has the biggest willy, as all hard-ons look the same. Thank god for BishUK.com, which answers those hideous questions you just can't ask your parents, like 'Can you break your penis?' or 'Is masturbation dangerous?' or 'Is there a maximum number of times you can ejaculate safely in a day?' We had the sex-ed talk at school, but it's all girl stuff, for boys it's just about how to put a condom on, and keep it on for ever and ever unless you want to get a girl pregnant. My mum has friends who can't pregnant so I know quite a lot about it as they talk all the time. I think being a sperm donor in the future would be good – helping lots of people to have children who really want them. I think I won't want children myself until I am at least 30 or 40, I definitely want to do lots of things before having to settle with one girlfriend.

9.1iii Martha, a new mum who conceived naturally

A little bit of background: I had had two doctors in my past tell me that it was unlikely I would ever get pregnant, or carry a baby to term – a combination of physiology and pathology apparently – so it was never really something I factored into my long term plans/future daydreams. It changed when I became pregnant at the wrong time, in the wrong lifetime, and it didn't leave by itself. It made the decision to terminate that little bit harder. Not that there's anything easy in such a decision.

And it was like a switch had flipped. Suddenly I was broody for the first time ever. And would cry over babies. Yes, grief was going on too, but so was something physical. My body *wanted* to be pregnant. What *turned me on* was the idea of getting knocked up. It was nuts.

Cue awesome guy. Ha! Be careful what you wish for!

Steve and I discussed children before we ever slept together – at my prompting, because I needed him to know that if a pregnancy did occur, I would not be terminating it, and he would be *a dad*. The previous pregnancy having been conceived whilst I was on the pill, I was very aware that that was what sex was really all about, and I didn't trust contraception to work. Plus he smelled right, like home.

He said he'd always imagined having two; but had given up on the idea that he would ever meet someone to have one with, let alone two, some years ago. I said that I'd not have another abortion, and that at some time in the future, I'd like to stop trying to prevent pregnancy.

We played with fire a couple of times, and caught fire. And now we have the most beautiful five-and-a-half-month-old boy.

And how is it being the mum of a small baby? Well, you know how everyone describes it as 'life changing'? Life changing ain't strong enough. For me, being the stay at home one, it has been Life Hijacking. I, me, Martha who was, does not exist anymore. She doesn't have time to. I celebrate if I can do the washing up now, let alone dye my hair. Hell, it's a good day if I run a brush though it!

I was on people's radars for Postnatal Depression because I had set it up so, given a long history of plain ol' regular depression. I skirted the edges of it certainly, and conversations with a great GP allowed me to realise I was not experiencing depression, but what he called Adjustment Crisis, and I called Grief. Grief for the life I had before. Grief for the life I will never live again. That clarity – naming it – made it easier to flow with. And Finn. Finn thawed my heart. He snuggled into the crook of my arm, with a full-belly face, and fell asleep, and I melted,

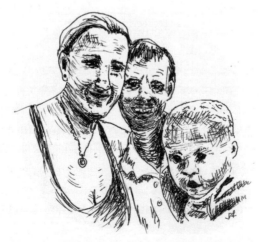

and stepped fully into my role now as Mummy. It will only be a short few years that I hold that role, before I become Muuu-uuum, and then he'll be off, finding his own life.

We were warned: 'It's the hardest job you'll ever do'. Yep. It is. In spades. And then he sleeps. And he is the most beautiful thing I've ever seen. And I'll stay up just those few minutes longer to watch him.

Up until he was eight weeks old, and had his first formula, every cell, every molecule of him, with the exception of one, right at the start, came from me. Oh. No. Wait. He breathed. Bum. I've just ruined the magic of that with facts. Me and the air.

People ask me can I imagine life without him now? Yes, I can imagine how life would be had he never have existed. It's pretty much Facebook and not much else. And unfortunately yes, I can imagine life without him now he does exist, and it's horrifying. It breaks my heart every time my brain takes me there – which, thanks to pregnancy re-wiring, it does with startling frequency. And every time results in another safety measure being put in place. For example, I now carry scissors in my glove box, in case the car flips into a deep water filled ditch and Finn is strapped into his car seat. The rest of the time I have to breathe the saying 'hold on tightly, let go lightly'. To every cuddle, to every set of clothes he outgrows, to every first, to every scream, to every smile.

Steve says I should mention self-belief. He says I should have greater self-belief after going through labour. This doesn't ring true for me, because I never doubted myself when facing or experiencing labour. I think it is more true to say that *he* has more belief in me since seeing me go through labour.

I went to sit by the ocean when I was pregnant and scared. I asked for The Sea to give me her counsel, and she told me, 'Yes, he will destroy you. He will also make you.' That's the truest truth I can give on it. It's Raw Love.

9.1iv Richard, a stepdad who conceived naturally

I thought I'd won the lottery when Amy was born. When I met Julie she had Lizzie, her five-year-old daughter, already and I loved her like my own. Conceiving quickly was brilliant – 'Super sperm!' joked Julie, as it had taken her a while to get pregnant before. Going through the pregnancy was amazing for us all as a family, we got a book looking at what was happening and paid to have 4D scans with a video. Confession – for a time it was my screensaver! We thought two children in the family was enough and weren't actively trying when we got pregnant again – we only really knew about being pregnant when Julie lost the baby at 10 weeks. We tried and tried again and this time it took about nine months to get pregnant and having lost a baby, the pregnancy was an anxious time, but when Blake was born with loads of hair it was like winning the lottery – again. The sperm might not be as super as was first thought, but we definitely don't want any more children. I'm planning to have a vasectomy so Julie doesn't have to take anything or use anything to stop getting pregnant again.

9.1v Clarissa, a mum who conceived with IVF using donor eggs and who would like more children

We tried to conceive naturally, but we had negative test after negative test and the most frustrating thing was there was apparently nothing wrong with either of us. So originally we said we'd just do three cycles of IVF, through the NHS. These were manageable and work and friends and family were supportive. After our third cycle was unsuccessful everyone thought that was it, we should be content and accept our lot and embrace adoption as a positive solution to becoming parents. But we went along to an information event and it only confirmed that adoption wasn't right for either of us. We tried to carry on, almost blot out all the treatment, all of the pain, but couldn't.

We saw an advert for a package deal where you had several cycles and your money was refunded if your treatment was not successful. We figured it would be a waste of money if we got pregnant first time, but if it took three cycles it would work out cheaper and if it wasn't successful, we could walk away without cost. It was almost too good to be true, and we had to be accepted, I suppose to see if we were in with a chance of success. The waiting to know if we'd been accepted was almost as stressful as treatment, but eventually we were. So we re-mortgaged without telling anyone – we couldn't cope with the looks of well-meaning parents.

We had three more cycles. Trying to not let work know was really exhausting; the medication this time felt more powerful, or I reacted with more intensity, but it was the two week waits that were the worst. I didn't know what to do – stay active, lie down? Was sex safe? Was having a big poo safe? Might I expel my embryos? Does anyone else have that thought? I thought I'd lost the plot! Sadly, yet again it didn't work, yet again we weren't ready to stop.

We found a clinic with an egg bank attached and had two more cycles. Thankfully property prices increased quicker than our wages, so we re-mortgaged again and thankfully – incredibly – the second cycle produced our daughter.

It makes me feel like an ungrateful sad old woman, but now I am desperate for another. I had hoped we'd have frozen embryos – or 'frosties' as they are sometimes called – but there were no spare embryos suitable to freeze.

My parents absolutely understand my desire for a second, my dad especially; I was their third and he shared quite happily that people thought they were mad having me back then, checking if they knew there was now contraception available. They are helping financially with our next cycle. I might be 50, but fertility, up to a point, is a bit more timeless these days if you can be comfortable with donor conception – and we very much are! We are so comfy if there are spare embryos this time and if it works, we might even have a third.

9.1vi Andrew, a father of twins conceived through IVF

You work hard and reap the rewards, that's how I operate, putting in the effort to appreciate and value the results. We've a lovely life, Sian and I. We met at uni, lived in a flat share, got married, bought a flat and then a house, waited until we could afford good childcare before starting to try for a baby. We then had sex to order dictated by the smiley face (honestly!) on the ovulation kit. We stopped coffee, stopped alcohol, stopped all things fun, cycling became a no-no, just in case it squashed my precious swimmers, restricting their tail-swishing abilities.

Then it was tests, tests and more tests, but apparently we were 'unexplained', the suggested option was IVF, it sounded

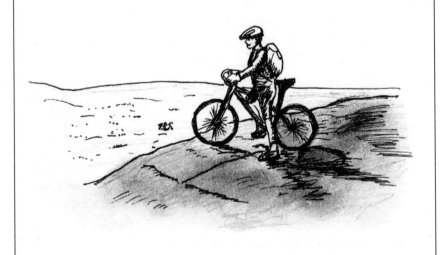

simple, but in reality – it's evil. Never mind my theories of working hard and reaping rewards, there's nothing you can do to help, you feel incompetent as well as impotent and giving the injections felt more like abuse, even though Sian wanted me to inject her. It was the one thing I could do, other than produce a sample, the 'walk of shame' through the clinic when you feel all eyes are on you. No pressure there then! The practical side was easier than feeling I should know how to support Sian more; in the end she said, 'Shut up and just be there for me!' so I made sure I went to every scan during our treatment. I was often the only man at the clinic, but I wanted to be there. The consultant let me push the plunger thing for the embryo transfer – it was amazing.

Any regrets? Well, we had twins from our first cycle which is wonderful but I might have wished we'd transferred one embryo to friends when they were smaller as it felt a lot to manage. Now I can escape on my bike when it gets a bit chaotic, there are no regrets. Might sound mad, but we've got six embryos in the freezer, and though I don't think we want six more children, we will definitely try for another in a few years. This time we will definitely just transfer one!

9.1vii Rachel, who ceased IVF and became a therapist

It was pouring with rain and I was standing in the doorway of the community hall where we had just had a party for my step-daughter's 14th birthday, when I had the realisation that if our third round of IVF was successful (slim chance) we could be doing this again in 15 years' time. That was the start of the end of our IVF journey and helped us make the very emotional decision not to do a third. At the same time, I had decided I wanted to do a Masters in Psychotherapy and we couldn't afford to do both.

That was seven years ago and I have never ever regretted that decision, in fact it was one of the best decisions of my life. I have an amazingly rewarding and fulfilling career as a psychotherapist in private practice. I have two incredible step-children and feel so fortunate to have very strong loving relationships with them both, and I know they have helped me to accept a future without my own children. Oh, and we got a crazy cocker spaniel puppy, who makes me laugh very single day.

9.1viii Anthony, one half of a fostering couple who have now adopted

I was going to co-parent with a lesbian friend in my late twenties, but she got into a new relationship and they decided they wanted a sperm bank donor, so that was me, ousted. I'd given up on the family man thing until I met Rob and he said he'd always wanted children and how were we going to go about that? No ifs, he just saw I was great with kids and assumed I was up for it too. We're both social workers, and though neither of us works with children we both have friends who do, and they suggested fostering; we did respite fostering with children with special needs for three years, just weekends and a few times over Christmas. We worked with each of the families for around a year, we could have carried on but by the end of the first year we knew we wanted our own family. We explored surrogacy but decided we wanted to be 'equal' parents and not one of us be a genetic parent and the other not. We stayed with our fostering agency who also do 'foster to adopt', so as well as being approved as foster carers we did extra work to be approved for adoption. When we started fostering Archie, we got to know his mum and he still sees her regularly even though legally he is now our son. Families are made, not born!

9.1ix Debi, who adopted after many attempts at IVF

While we were doing IVF, I asked Colin, my husband, 'When do we stop?' After six fresh cycles, two frozen cycles, a second ectopic pregnancy (which should never happen with IVF, and I'd had one trying to conceive naturally), and finally a miscarriage a week before Christmas, I told Colin that sadly I had had enough... My body and my heart couldn't take any more. After selling our house to help fund our heartbreak, I now knew it was time to stop and look at other ways to become parents.

We applied for adoption in February 2002 and it was a very long, hard, intrusive process. If you have any skeletons then they need to know them. I struggled with discussing my first marriage breakdown, as it was because he didn't want kids... After a year focusing so intensely on it, I admitted to having become depressed and put it on hold for a year and a half. Once I was in a better place, we continued. We had meetings with social workers almost weekly for about six months – it was hard trying to act 'happy' and 'normal' and show 'how

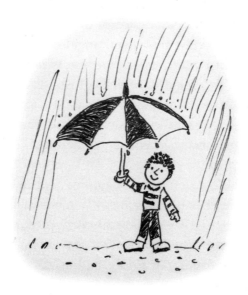

much in love' we were. For months it was like 'Look, we are a fab couple who will give a fab home to a poor baby'. So once you're accepted, which includes a meeting in a big room with social workers, doctors, judges etc throwing you crazy 'what if' questions, you are in limbo... waiting... waiting... waiting.... Finally, after 13 months, we got THE CALL!!! I was in work and can't remember how I got home!!! Our social worker brought another social worker whose first words were 'So Dennon is 23 months old' and I had to ask 'Is it a boy or a girl?' She said, 'It's a boy...' and my heart flipped out!!!!! She had no pictures but arranged for yet another meeting.

At the meeting I cried, and at the same time I couldn't stop grinning. We met Dennon's foster parents who gave us a photo album. My God – my son was beautiful! (I was scared he would be ugly). The very first picture I saw, he was wearing a little light blue waistcoat at a wedding and I fell in love. From then on it was a whirlwind. Arranging adoption leave from work – it's the same as maternity leave, so I had a year off – then arranging our two week 'Get to know Dennon' before he came to live with us. We had a final meeting, then we were taken to see him. I cannot express my excitement enough. When we got to the door it was opened and this little blonde, blue eyed angel of a child said 'Hi...' We had bought a build a bear for him which barked 'I love you'. 'Bertie', he called it, after his foster family's dog, and he loved it. We took him to the park and that first day he said 'Dad' to Colin. My husband was so proud! Two days later he said 'Mummy' and my heart was complete. That first year was the best year of my life.

Jump to 2017, and Dennon is almost 11. I can honestly say that whilst there have been times I questioned myself as a parent and times I've wished I hadn't adopted, that was when my depression returned and with it panic attacks and anxiety. Now it's just 'normal', in a good but level way. Dennon is a beautiful, healthy, loving young man, who has his moments like any other child. Occasionally he tries our patience, but if asked 'Would I do it again?' I would say, 'I wish I had done it twice and got my son a sister or a brother.'

9.1x Tracey, who adopted, fostered and also works as a counsellor

When we adopted, life was incredibly difficult. We had no support, which left us exhausted as parents. At the same time I was asked to attend a 'fun weekend' organised by a group of former Fertility Network UK members who had formed a support section of the charity for people who were involuntarily childless. I was going along to find out how clinics could better support people who left without a baby – should counselling be available at the clinic, or did people want to 'run to the hills'?

I arrived to find everyone was getting to know each other, no one was asking 'how many children have you got?' or questioning why you didn't have any. There was one marquee for people to camp, another for partying. No one wanted to be there – in that that they had all wanted children – but here was a safe environment, where no one was judged. Momentarily I wondered how our life might have been if we'd been turned down for adoption. Could we have looked that happy? I was – thankfully! – having counselling at the time, as it was the topic I came back to for months. How did I know we'd done the right thing?

I know now that there *isn't* a right thing, just decisions made that feel more right than other options. There isn't an easy path for anyone struggling to conceive but there are lots of different possibilities and these days there is plenty of support out there, whichever route you take.

9.2 Making friends with *your* fertility

'In every parting there is an image of death.'
George Eliot

Throughout this book we've talked often about the importance of accepting loss, and, as the stories in this chapter illustrate so powerfully, it's evident that fertility – our ability to procreate, or not – can bring great sorrow as well as joy.

My own experience of anxiety and depression has taught me how helpful it can be to acknowledge and give space to the difficult and darker aspects of ourselves because fighting or denying them doesn't serve us in the long run. But **whatever happens to us in terms of having or not having children,** alongside acknowledging loss, **it's also hugely important to be kind to ourselves**. It's this ability to nurture and look after ourselves – our *whole* selves, mind, body and spirit – that lies at the heart of the 'making friends' ethos. The title of our book reflects the belief that **it's helpful to be your own best friend, taking care of and being responsible for yourself.**

I certainly don't want to suggest you view your own experiences through rose-tinted glasses, but I'd like to propose that **if we see our journey through our fertile years as an ever-shifting and ongoing period of psychological and spiritual *transformation*, then it's much easier to reframe it as a positive – or, more accurately, multifaceted – experience.** Arguably, it's more helpful to view our fertility this way than to see it as rigidly subdivided into separate chunks – puberty/pregnancy/parenthood etc – even though that's what we've done with our chapter headings in this book. Otherwise it's so easy to berate ourselves for not meeting up to our own internal standards – we've not become pregnant in the time we envisaged, we're not the parents we think we should be, we ought to adopt if our IVF has failed, yadda yadda. With this rigid view and life mapped out this tightly, we end up forever comparing ourselves with our peers and our own internalized ideals, measuring ourselves up against imaginary timetables and finding ourselves wanting.

How much easier it is to be a good friend to yourself if you are more forgiving and accepting than that! I'm reminded again of that FLO string, how flexible it was, and how fluid our emotions are, and of how Tracey wrote of allowing our plans to be written in pencil, not etched in stone. I'll return to the situation that I touched upon in Chapter 8, to illustrate.

Having come to terms with not having my own children – insofar as one ever can – I met Tom when I was 44, and he had a son, Sebastian, who was eight at the time. Tom and I are now married, and over the last ten years Seb has spent a lot of time with us, and we've had – and continue to have – a lot of fun together (as well as some almighty rows). I'm very aware that being a stepmother is not the same as being his mother; Seb already *has* a mum, and they are very close. (My own parents both remarried and I know how galling it is when people assume your stepparents are your parents – it used to make me squirm.) Nonetheless our unique and part-time family is like one of the chocolates Tracey made sound so appetising earlier in this book. It satisfies some of my nurturing capacity and is a big and important part of my life. It's as Rebecca said in Chapter 5: in the moment that I surrendered control and let go, something arrived. The experience taught me to accept what lies beyond my control, to be flexible and to trust the bigger picture.

> *'Life is what happens when you are busy making other plans.'*
> **John Lennon**

9.3 Beyond fertility – where now?

It might seem a strange note to end on, but I'd like to include **a very gentle reminder that there is more to life – as in the whole beginning-to-end of life – than babies.** In time every woman ceases to be naturally fertile, and a massive drop in oestrogen levels will affect every part of her body, including her brain. At this point women cease menstruating and go through the menopause (a subject explored in much detail in the sister book to this one, *Making Friends with the Menopause*). Men don't have such a brutal wake-up call in this regard as their fertility declines more gradually, although sperm quality and testosterone levels decrease with age, making it harder to father children as you get older.

But instead of resenting men for having greater longevity in terms of their fertility, perhaps it's better – more empowering – for women to embrace what our more clearly delineated window bestows. That women experience the menopause can also mean that we are more able to appreciate the transient nature of being. After all, **that we're no longer able to give life is a stark reminder that we are going to die**. Add to this the fact that invariably – even if we conceive later on using donor eggs and/or sperm – babies become children who become adults, and at a certain point, if you've had them, they will (with a few exceptions), leave home. This can give focus and open up opportunity, allowing you to find a new space in which to **create what it means to be 'you' in the middle years of your life**. The same is true for fathers when children fly the nest, and (together or separately) there can be new and exciting roads to explore that draw upon your capacity for nurturing.

This has been the case for me. I'm not the first to make a connection between giving birth and writing, and whilst I think drawing a parallel between authoring and mothering often fails to

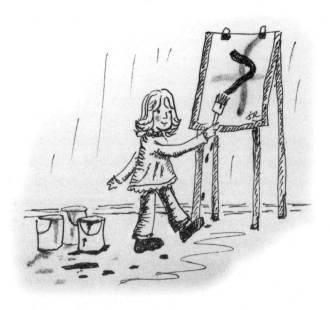

convey fully what it takes to be either, I'm aware that I put a lot of my nurturing capacity into my work. It's no coincidence I've a creative job – it satisfies a big part of me. But lately I'm aware that I've been doing a different kind of creative work. I'm no longer in advertising, and now, being a publisher as well as a writer, it allows me to nurture other people – including those new to the book-writing adventure like Tracey – as well as myself.

I'm more interested in building a community and support, so in that regard I'm less go-getting. This book is one example of my personal shift in focus, but it certainly wasn't something I planned to write back when I was 21, imagining my future. It's something that evolved; something that feels right to do at this point in time. In that respect it underlines the ancient wisdom that **the moment to focus on is now.**

9.4 And so, the end is here

Online, in newspapers, on TV and from doctors and consultants – much of what we hear about fertility and infertility sits firmly within a western scientific and medical tradition. The danger with this is we can end up ignoring the more nebulous but no less vital impact of the unconscious, and fail to consider our minds and bodies together, holistically. In *Making Friends with your Fertility* we've tried to balance these out. At times, yes, we've been logical – neither Tracey nor I see rationality as unhelpful – and we have included a fair amount of basic biology, particularly in the early chapters. But we've also given space to consider emotional responses and an alternative point of view.

Tracey and I are two very different people and naturally don't agree on everything, but we do agree that **it's awareness that matters. In order to make a successful passage through puberty, our fertile years and beyond, we need to be *aware* of what is happening to us**. Just as a young girl might be frightened if she doesn't know why there is blood between her legs, a young man might be fearful of his penis falling off. Equally, a middle-aged woman may be trepidatious if she doesn't understand the menopausal phenomenon, and an older man may balk at examining his testicles, anxious about what he might find there.

In this book we've endeavoured to take some of this fear of the unknown away. We haven't dealt with every issue, we simply don't have the space, and we're not experts in every area, so we've had to be selective, and paint with a broad brush. What we've aimed to do is give an overview, and we hope that as you near the last page, you have found this perspective helpful. Fertility, families, marriage, singledom, motherhood, fatherhood, being child free, the menopause, old age and dying… we each have to find our own path, but knowledge is power, and the support and wisdom of others can help illuminate the way.

'You only have one life, but if you do it right, once is enough.'
Mae West

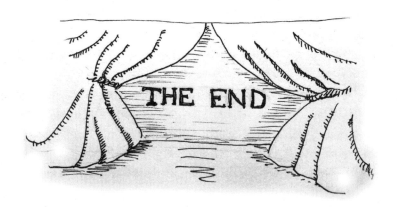

JOIN THE CONVERSATION

'Never doubt that a small group of thoughtful, committed citizens can change the world. Indeed, it is the only thing that ever has.'
Margaret Mead

Time and again throughout this book we've heard others say that talking about what you're experiencing can lighten the load and increase understanding, and hearing from others who've been through something similar can provide reassurance that you're not alone. Tracey and I hope that's part of what this book, *Making Friends with your Fertility*, with its interjections and insights from many throughout, has given you.

If you'd like to continue the conversation yourself, why not join the **Facebook group** we've often mentioned? It's called *Making Friends with your Fertility* and

www.facebook.com/groups/makingfriendswithyourfertility/

is the place to go in order to share tips and seek advice from others too. If you'd prefer not to, that's fine. Tracey and I would like to end by saying **thank you** for reading.

AN EXPLANATION OF ACRONYMS
ASSOCIATED WITH FERTILITY

2WW = Two week wait
A/F = Aunt Flo (period)
AH = Assisted hatching
AMH = Anti mullerian hormone
ART = Assisted reproductive technique
BCP = Birth control pills
BET = Blastocyst embryo transfer
BFN = Big fat negative
BFP = Big fat positive
BICA = British Infertility Counselling
 Association
CD = Cycle day
CM = Cervical mucus
DE = Donor eggs
DHEA = Dehydroepiandrosterone
DI = Donor insemination
DD = Darling daughter
DH = Darling husband
DPO = Days post-ovulation
DPR = Days post-retrieval
DP = Darling partner
DPT = Days post-transfer
DS = Darling son
DS = Donor sperm
DW = Darling wife
EC = Egg collection
EDD = Estimated due date
ENDO = Endometriosis
ERPC = Evacuation of retained products
 of conception
ET = Embryo transfer
EWCM = Egg white cervical mucus
FER = Frozen embryo replacement
FET = Frozen embryo transfer
FP = Follicular phase
FSH = Follicle stimulating hormone
H/B = Heartbeat
HCG = Human chorionic gonadotropin
HFEA = Human Fertilisation &
 Embryology Authority
HPT = Home pregnancy test
HRT = Hormone replacement therapy
HSC = Hysteroscopy
HSG = Hysterosalpingogram
ICSI = Intra-cytoplasmic sperm injection

IMHO = In my humble opinion
IMO = In my opinion
FNUK = Fertility Network UK
IPS = Intended Parents (Surrogacy)
IUI = Intra-uterine insemination
IVF = In vitro fertilisation
IYKWIM = If you know what I mean
LAP = Laparoscopy
LH = Luteinising hormone
LMP = Last menstrual period
LP = Luteal phase
LPD = Luteal phase defect
MA = Miscarriage association
M/C = Miscarriage
MESA = Microsurgical epididymal sperm
 aspiration
M/W = Midwife
OD = Ovum Donor (Egg Donor)
ODR = Ovum Donor Recipient (Egg
 Donor Recipient)
OI = Ovulation induction
OS = Ovum Sharer (Egg sharer/donor)
OV = Ovulation
OHSS = Ovarian hyperstimulation
 syndrome
OPK = Ovulation predictor kit
PCO = Polycystic ovaries
PCOS = Polycystic ovary syndrome
PESA Percutaneous epididymal sperm
 aspiration
PG = Pregnant
PID = Pelvic inflammatory disease
PMS = Pre-menstrual syndrome
POF = Premature ovarian failure
PUPO = Pregnant until proven othewise
SA = Sperm or Semen analysis
SANDS = Stillbirth and Neonatal Death
 Society
S/B Stillbirth
SI = Secondary infertility
STD = Sexually transmitted disease
TESA = Testicular sperm aspiration
TTC = Trying to conceive
U/S = Ultrasound

NOTES

1   http://www.independent.co.uk/news/science/sperm-count-west-men-health-drop-60-per-cent-years-modern-life-a7859491.html

2   http://www.bbc.co.uk/science/0/21755753

3   https://www.amazon.co.uk/Two-Week-Wait-Sarah-Rayner/dp/0330544101/ref=tmm_pap_swatch_0?_encoding=UTF8&qid=&sr=,

4.   There are fertility hormones that a GP can test, some that are usually only performed in secondary care and others that are often only discovered once assistance to try to conceive is needed.

5   https://www.fertility authority.com/trouble-conceiving-and-infertility/premature-ovarian-aging-poa/premature-ovarian-aging-poa-can-it-be

6   I would love to be able to state factually that DHEA might improve fertility, or even give a boost to our desire, but there is more research needed.

7   https://www.fertility authority.com/trouble-conceiving-and-infertility/premature-ovarian-aging-poa/premature-ovarian-aging-poa-can-it-be

8   A urologist is a specialist in the urinary tract and male reproductive organs. https://www.healthcareers.nhs.uk/explore-roles/surgery/urology

9   http://www.nature.com/ijir/journal/v15/n1/full/3900945a.html

10   www.endometriosis-uk.org

11   http://www.nhs.uk/Conditions/Periods/Pages/Introduction.aspx#Sanitary products

12   There is the advice about how to keep your cup clean here: http://metro.co.uk/2017/07/06/menstrual-cups-are-more-likely-to-cause-toxic-shock-syndrome-than-tampons-claims-study-6758784/

13   http://www.nhs.uk/Livewell/menopause/Pages/Prematuremenopause.aspx

14   https://www.daisynetwork.org.uk/
15   https://blogs.scientificamerican.com/bering-in-mind/why-do-human-testicles-hang-like-that/
16   https://www.ovulationcalculator.com/journey-of-sperm/
17   https://www.livescience.com/23845-sexy-swimmers-sperm-facts.html
18   https://en.oxforddictionaries.com/definition/sexual_intercourse
19   John Keay (2010). *India: A History: from the Earliest Civilisations to the Boom of the Twenty-first Century.* Grove Press. pp. 81–103.
20   https://cks.nice.org.uk/infertility#!scenario:1
      https://www.nice.org.uk/guidance/cg156/resources/cg156-fertility-full-guideline3 Page 68 section 5.3
21   http://www.sciencedirect.com/science/article/pii/S0003347213002121
      https://www.ncbi.nlm.nih.gov/pmc/articles/PMC5087695/
22   http://www.nhs.uk/conditions/vaginismus/pages/introduction.aspx
      http://www.nhs.uk/conditions/vaginismus/pages/introduction.aspx
23   http://www.nhs.uk/conditions/ejaculation-problems/Pages/Introduction.aspx
      http://www.nhs.uk/conditions/ejaculation-problems/Pages/Introduction.aspx
24   https://www.thestorkconception.co.uk/
25   http://www.bounty.com/about-bounty/bounty-packs/pregnancy-information-pack
26   http://www.bbc.co.uk/schools/gcsebitesize/science/add_ocr_pre_2011/growth_development/singlecellrev1.shtml
27   http://www.bounty.com/getting-pregnant/getting-pregnant-naturally/am-i-pregnant/implantation-bleeding
28   http://www.nhs.uk/Conditions/pregnancy-and-baby/Pages/dating-scan-ultrasound-10-11-12-13-weeks-pregnant.aspx
29   https://www.nct.org.uk/
30   https://www.amazon.com/Prenatal-Development-Parents-Lived-Experiences/dp/0393711064
31   http://www.pandasfoundation.org.uk/
32   http://www.pandasfoundation.org.uk/
33   http://www.nhs.uk/conditions/pregnancy-and-baby/pages/where-can-i-give-birth.aspx

34   http://www.netdoctor.co.uk/conditions/pregnancy-and-family/a9120/childbirth-8211-what-are-your-options/

35   https://www.dogstrust.org.uk/help-advice/FACTsheets-downloads/FACTsheetnewbabynov13.pdf
      https://www.bluecross.org.uk/pet-advice/your-cat-and-your-baby

36   http://www.expressyourselfmums.co.uk/hospital-grade-rental-breastpumps

37   https://www.amazon.com/Confessions-Other-Mother-Non-Biological-Lesbian/dp/0807079634/

38   http://www.nhs.uk/news/2016/07July/Pages/Pregnancy-supplements-dont-help-just-take-vit-D-and-folic-acid.aspx

39   http://www.nhs.uk/chq/Pages/2319.aspx

40   http://www.everydayhealth.com/atrial-fibrillation/living-with/this-is-your-heart-on-energy-drinks/

41   http://www.nhs.uk/news/2016/07July/Pages/Pregnancy-supplements-dont-help-just-take-vit-D-and-folic-acid.aspx

42   https://www.thoughtco.com/immune-system-372421

43   http://www.livestrong.com/article/550339-does-pineapple-juice-help-the-lining-of-the-uterus/

44   http://www.nhs.uk/Livewell/loseweight/Pages/BodyMassIndex.aspx

45   http://www.fertilityfriends.co.uk/f
      https://healthunlocked.com/fertility-network-uk

46   http://www.nhs.uk/news/2016/07July/Pages/Pregnancy-supplements-dont-help-just-take-vit-D-and-folic-acid.aspx

47   http://www.fertstert.org/article/S0015-0282(13)02998-1/abstract
      https://www.ncbi.nlm.nih.gov/pubmed/23823924

48   http://principal6fertility.com/wp-content/uploads/2015/04/DHEA-1.pdf

49   https://www.ntnu.edu/news/hard-workouts-reduced-fertility

50   https://www.ncbi.nlm.nih.gov/pmc/articles/PMC3733210/

51   https://www.ncbi.nlm.nih.gov/pubmed/20098228

52   http://www.nhs.uk/Livewell/fitness/Pages/pilates.aspx

53   http://www.nhs.uk/Livewell/fitness/Pages/pilates.aspx

54   https://www.headspace.com/blog/2014/11/19/walk-into-a-mindful-moment/

https://louiseannwilson.com/projects/warnscale It might be for everyone, but this walk, written as an art project around childlessness and infertility, might pique your interest if you're a regular hiker.

55   https://www.borrowmydoggy.com/

56   http://www.webmd.com/balance/guide/what-is-holistic-medicine#1

57   http://www.professionalstandards.org.uk/what-we-do/accredited-registers/find-a-register

58   https://www.cnhc.org.uk/

59   https://www.acupuncture.org.uk/

60   http://www.verity-pcos.org.uk/

61   http://www.acupuncture-fertility.org

62   http://www.atcm.co.uk/

63   https://reproductivereflexologists.org/

64   https://www.miscarriageassociation.org.uk/information/miscarriage/

65   http://www.nhs.uk/Conditions/Miscarriage/Pages/Causes.aspx

66   http://www.nhs.uk/Conditions/miscarriage/Pages/Introduction.aspx

67   In the future it may be more common to use three: https://www.newscientist.com/article/2107219-exclusive-worlds-first-baby-born-with-new-3-parent-technique/

68   http://myfuturefamily.org.uk/ https://www.fertilityshow.co.uk/

69   http://www.nataliegambleassociates.co.uk/

70   http://www.nataliegambleassociates.co.uk/

71   https://www.stonewall.org.uk

72   http://www.prideangel.com/
      http://www.bica.net/
      http://www.nationalfertilitysociety.co.uk/

73   http://www.who.int/reproductivehealth/topics/infertility/definitions/en/

74   http://www.nhs.uk/conditions/infertility/pages/diagnosis.aspx

75   http://www.nhs.uk/Conditions/Infertility/Pages/Treatment.aspx

76   http://www.nhs.uk/Conditions/Infertility/Pages/Treatment.aspx

77   http://www.nhs.uk/Conditions/Fibroids/Pages/Introduction.aspx

78 http://www.nhs.uk/conditions/hysteroscopy/pages/introduction
.aspx

79 http://www.nhs.uk/Conditions/Endometriosis/Pages/Introduction
.aspx

80 I feel this is a more appropriate point for a sperm test. I checked on
the NHS website and it seems GPs will refer men for them.

81 http://fertilitynetworkuk.org/

82 https://www.nice.org.uk/guidance/cg156

83 http://www.fertilityfairness.co.uk/

84 http://fertilitynetworkuk.org/wp-
content/uploads/2016/10/FACTSHEET-Choosing-a-Fertility-
Clinic-October-2016.pdf

85 http://fertilitynetworkuk.org/wp-
content/uploads/2016/10/FACTSHEET-Choosing-a-Fertility-
Clinic-October-2016.pdf

86 http://www.hfea.gov.uk/

87 https://beta.hfea.gov.uk/code-of-practice/

88 www.hfea.gov.uk

89 You'll find a list of them at the end back of this book.

90 http://fertilitynetworkuk.org/
http://www.hfea.gov.uk

91 http://www.webmd.com/balance/guide/ayurvedic-treatments

92 https://www.nice.org.uk/guidance/cg156/ifp/chapter/intrauterine
-insemination

93 www.bica.net

94 In the UK it is only legal to fertilize mature eggs.

95 https://www.hfea.gov.uk/treatments/fertility-
preservation/embryo-freezing/

96 http://www.progress.org.uk/home

97 https://www.verywell.com/what-is-interpersonal-neurobiology-
2337621

98 http://books.wwnorton.com/books/Prenatal-Development-and-
Parents-Lived-Experiences

99 http://www.tangledwebs.org.uk/tw/

100 http://www.hfea.gov.uk/

101 https://www.ngdt.co.uk/

102 https://www.dcnetwork.org/

103 http://www.brilliantbeginnings.co.uk/

104 https://www.surrogacyuk.org/

105 https://www.surrogacy.org.uk/

106 http://www.telegraph.co.uk/news/health/11760004/Louise-Brown-the-first-IVF-baby-reveals-family-was-bombarded-with-hate-mail.html

107 http://ifqtesting.blob.core.windows.net/umbraco-website/1783/fertility-treatment-2014-trends-and-figures.pdf page 4 Taken from HFEA 2014 results – 1 2015 update has not been made(!) http://ifqtesting.blob.core.windows.net/umbraco-website/1783/fertility-treatment-2014-trends-and-figures.pdf page 4

108 http://www.resolve.org/family-building-options/ivf-art/what-are-my-chances-of-success-with-ivf.html?referrer=https://www.google.co.uk/

109 http://www.bounty.com/getting-pregnant/getting-pregnant-naturally/am-i-pregnant/implantation-bleeding

110 http://www.webmd.boots.com/pregnancy/guide/chemical-pregnancy and http://www.huffingtonpost.co.uk/dee-armstrong/what-exactly-is-a-chemica_b_5834130.html

111 https://www.rcog.org.uk/en/patients/patient-leaflets/recovering-from-surgical-management-of-a-miscarriage/

112 https://www.miscarriageassociation.org.uk/

113 'As many as one in seven couples' http://www.motherandbaby.co.uk/trying-for-a-baby/pregnancy-planning/fertility-conditions-and-treatment/secondary-infertility

114 secondaryinfertilityuk@gmail.com

115 https://www.pms.org.uk/

116 https://www.mind.org.uk/about-us/local-minds/resilience

117 https://psychcentral.com/lib/what-is-a-trigger/

118 http://www.fertilitynetworkuk.org

119 http://www.nfaw.org.uk/

120 www.bica.net

121 https://www.quora.com/What-are-the-archetypes-of-femininity-1

122 https://bemindful.co.uk/

123 https://www.mind.org.uk/information-support/drugs-and-treatments/cognitive-behavioural-therapy-cbt/#.WSmT0mjyuUk

124 https://www.mind.org.uk/information-support/drugs-and-treatments/dialectical-behaviour-therapy-dbt/#.WSmT12jyuUk

125 http://www.nhs.uk/Conditions/stress-anxiety-depression/pages/mindfulness.aspx

126 http://www.nfaw.org.uk/wp-content/uploads/2015/06/When1+1doesnotmake2INUKinfoOct15.pdf

127 http://fertilitynetworkuk.org/for-those-trying-to-become-parents/support/fertility-groups/

128 www.bica.net

129 http://fertilitynetworkuk.org/for-those-facing-the-challenges-of-childlessness/information/ending-fertility-treatment/

130 https://www.sayinggoodbye.org/services/

131 http://www.gilltunstallcounselling.co.uk/east-london/14/Group-Counselling/Give-Sorrow-Words---Memorial-Ceremony.html

132 https://www.princes-trust.org.uk/support-our-work/volunteer/mentor

133 http://www.hft.org.uk/Get-involved/Volunteer/Ways-to-volunteer/Buddying/

134 http://www.befriending.co.uk/aboutbefriending.php

135 https://do-it.org/

136 www.bica.net

137 http://www.first4adoption.org.uk/

138 http://www.icacentre.org.uk/

139 https://www.adoptionuk.org/

140 https://www.thefosteringnetwork.org.uk/

141 http://www.hmrc.gov.uk/courses/syob3/fc/index.htm

142 http://fertilitynetworkuk.org/for-those-facing-the-challenges-of-childlessness/support/
     http://gateway-women.com/
     https://awoc.org/statisics/

143 http://www.childfree.net/
     https://www.childfreewomen.co.uk/

USEFUL WEBSITES

Medical
www.nhs.uk/Livewell/Fertility
www.rcog.org.uk
www.hfea.gov.uk
www.patient.info
www.bionews.org.uk

Support
www.fertilitynetworkuk.org
www.daisynetwork.org.uk
www.verity-pcos.org.uk
www.dcnetwork.org
www.pandasfoundation.org.uk
www.ngdt.co.uk
www.mensfe.net

Counselling
www.bica.net
www.cosrt.org.uk
www.relate.org.uk

Sexual Health
www.sexualadviceassociation.co.uk
www.bishuk.com

Pregnancy Loss
www.miscarriageassociation.org.uk

Menopause
www.menopausematters.co.uk
www.menopausesupport.co.uk

RECOMMENDED READING

The Period Book: A Girl's Guide to Growing Up,
   Karen Gravelle

Natural Solutions To Infertility: How to increase your chances of conceiving and preventing miscarriage,
   Marilyn Glenville

Eat Yourself Pregnant: Essential Recipes for Boosting Your Fertility Naturally,
   Zita West

The Day-by-Day Pregnancy Book: Comprehensive Advice from a Team of Experts and Amazing Images Every Single Day,
   Maggie Blott

Pregnancy for Men: The whole nine months,
   Mark Woods

Get A Life: His & Hers Survival Guide to IVF,
   Rosie Bray & Richard Mackney

Precious Babies: Pregnancy, birth and parenting after infertility,
   Kate Brian

Pride and Joy: A Guide for Lesbian, Gay, Bisexual and Trans Parents,
   Sarah Hagger-Holt & Rachel Hagger-Holt

Knock Yourself Up: No Man? No Problem?
   Louise Sloane

Prenatal Development and Parents' Lived Experiences: How Early Events Shape Our Psychophysiology and Relationships,
   Ann Diamond Weinstein & Michael Shea

The Pursuit of Motherhood,
   Jessica Hepburn

Donor Conception for Life: Psychoanalytic Reflections on New Ways of Conceiving,
   Katherine Fine

Silent Sorority: A Barren Woman Gets Busy, Angry, Lost and Found,
   Pamela Mahoney Tsigdinos

Living the Life Unexpected: 12 Weeks to Your Plan B for a Meaningful and Fulfilling Future Without Children,
   Jody Day

The Adoption Experience: Families Who Give Children a Second Chance,
   Ann Morris

Sarah's author website
www.sarah-rayner.com

ABOUT THE AUTHORS

Sarah Rayner

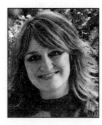

Sarah Rayner is the author of five novels including the international bestseller, *One Moment, One Morning* and the two follow-ups, *The Two Week Wait* and *Another Night, Another Day*.

Friendship is a theme common to Sarah's novels, and her non-fiction titles too. In 2014 she published *Making Friends with Anxiety, a warm, supportive little book to help ease worry and panic*. This was followed by a series of books including *Making Friends with the Menopause* and *Making Peace with Depression*. In 2017 Sarah set up the small press, creativepumpkinpublishing.com.

Sarah lives in Brighton with her husband, Tom, and stepson, Seb. You can hook up with her on **Facebook**, on **Twitter** and via her author website, **www.sarah-rayner.com**, where you can sign up for her mailing list and to receive her *Making Friends* magazine with a free short story and mood-boosting guide.

Tracey Sainsbury
AMBICA, Acc NCS, RMBACP

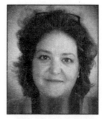

Tracey is a Senior Fertility Counsellor working with the London Women's Clinic Group. She has over 20 years' experience of volunteering and working professionally with fertility-related charities and organisations providing support, advice and information to people exploring their fertility.

Tracey lives in Wales with her husband Jonathan and is blessed, thanks to adoption, with their son, Lewis. You can follow Tracey on Twitter @IVFcounsellor and get in touch via the Facebook group, Making Friends with your Fertility.

London Women's Clinic

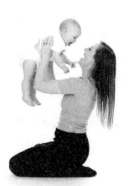

The London Women's Clinic was established in 1985 in Harley Street and went on to pioneer many of the techniques now routinely used in the treatment of infertility. Throughout this time our objective has always been treatment which is safe, effective and affordable. At the LWC you'll find:

- **Clinics across most regions of the UK** making access to treatment as easy as possible.

- **Caring, highly experienced staff**
  Our consultants and nursing staff have extensive experience in the treatment of infertility. In addition, we offer free monthly support groups, trained counsellors and fertility coaches for all our patients.

- **Minimum waiting times for treatment**
  We rarely have waiting lists for treatment. Treatment can thus start within six weeks or less meaning that when time is of the essence there are no unnecessary delays.

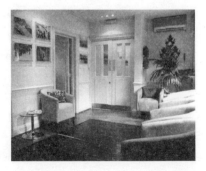

- **Excellent success rates**

  Whether from IVF or ICSI, egg donation or donor insemination, our results compare with the very best found in Britain.

- **Personalised approach**

  Our consultants will design a personal treatment plan based on your own fertility status, medical history and preferred treatment routes, with the single aim of maximising your chances of success.

- **Low cost packages and money-back guarantee in some of our regions**

  A number of our clinics are able to offer low cost packages of three cycles of treatment. Some may also offer a money-back guarantee if you meet their eligibility criteria and treatment is not successful.

- **Access to the largest sperm and egg banks in the UK**

  This usually means no wait for treatment with donor eggs or sperm. The London Women's Clinic patients have access to the largest catalogues of sperm and egg donors in the UK.

- **Treatment available to NHS patients**

  The LWC provides NHS-funded treatment to patients in selected areas of the country, including Bristol and the East of England. Contact us to find out more.

If you think fertility treatments are for you, we'd love to hear from you. You'll find the addresses of our clinics overleaf.

Londonwomensclinic.com

London Harley Street

113-115 Harley St, Marylebone, London W1G 6AP

+44 (0) 20 7563 4309

London Bridge

One St Thomas Street, London Bridge, London SE1 9RY

+44 (0) 20 7563 4309

Harrow

BMI The Clementine Churchill, Sudbury Hill, Harrow, HA1 3RX

+44 (0) 20 7563 4309

Cardiff

15 Windsor Pl, Cardiff CF10 3BY

+44 (0) 2920 236 301

Swansea

Ethos Building, Kings Rd, Swansea SA1 8AS

+44 (0) 1792 644 918

Darlington

Woodlands Hospital, Morton Park, Darlington DL1 4PL

+44 (0)1325 371 070

Essex - Brentwood Hospital

Brentwood Hospital, Shenfield Road, Brentwood, CM15 8EH

+44 (0) 1277 289 401

Kent

72 St. Dunstans St, Canterbury CT2 8BL

+44 (0) 1227 208 158

Bristol

2 Clifton Park, Bristol BS8 3BS

+44 (0) 117 906 4277